Here's what they're saying about
Low-Fat Living for Real People...

"An essential purchase [for core library collections] because of the ___ techniques and health facts."

"A book about healthy food that is as intriguing as a mystery nov___
Th___ ___nce Ledger (NJ)

"...a funny book with a serious purpose ... useful [in] a health crisis [or to] simply lower fat in diets."
The Philadelphia Daily News

"...educate[s] laypeople on making sound nutrition decisions that will stay with them for a lifetime."
The American Dietetic Association

"...brings us up-to-date with recipes and pragmatic (sometimes even humorous) advice on how to eat, shop and — yes — *live* low-fat."
Publishers Weekly

"[Leaves] the hard-to-read, even harder-to-understand nutrition books behind ... a user-friendly guide to transforming fatty diets into lean, mean menus."
The Times (Trenton, NJ)

"...highly recommended for individuals and families beginning the process of dietary change."
Topics in Clinical Nutrition

"...The authors have remembered...real people with real appetites, needing clearly written, reader-friendly information...they have stepped up to the plate and delivered."
Plano Star Courier (Texas)

"...one of the best books I have seen on heart-healthy eating and living."
Lake Worth Herald (Florida)

"...an exceptionally informative, easy-to-understand book dealing with diet modification."
The News Herald (Detroit)

"...filled with practical ideas and recipes spiced with innovation and individuality."
Lakewood Newspapers (Chicago)

LOW-FAT LIVING
for REAL PEOPLE

The Fat-Free Chocolate-Covered
Creme-Filled Mini-Cakes Diet
and Other Confusions of Low-Fat Eating
❧ EXPLAINED ❧

BY
LINDA LEVY
AND
FRANCINE GRABOWSKI, M.S., R.D.
CENTER FOR HEALTH & WELLNESS, COOPER HEALTH SYSTEM,
CHERRY HILL, NEW JERSEY

Drawings by **LINDA LEVY**

SECOND EDITION

Lake Isle Press, Inc. / New York

Library of Congress Catalogue Card Number: 97-75607
ISBN: 0-9627403-9-X

Book design: Christopher Kalb
Cover design: Karen Katz

January 1998
10 9 8 7 6 5 4 3 2 1

First Edition, 1994
Second Edition, 1998

For Paul,
who gave up tiramisù
– L.L.

For Tony, who gives his love,
energy, good nature, and music
– F.G.

Contents

Contents

Acknowledgments

This is a new edition, which brings with it new people to thank, and others to thank again.

Marlene Ciechoski, Shelly Margolis, and Jo Brozoski, women of heart; Princeton Public Library, Chilmark Public Library, and Corriel Library of the University of Medicine and Dentistry of New Jersey, whose reference staffs were invaluable; Dr. M. Kyu Chung and the Department of Family Medicine at Cooper Hospital, whose members provided vision and support. We thank our parents, Julius and Julia, John and Jane; our children, Jeff, Valerie, Deborah, Clare, Tim, and, of course, Charlie; Theresa, Anthony, Michael, Jennifer, Troy, and Leigh-Golding. And finally we thank Lake Isle Press and Hiroko Kiiffner, who said, the first time she met us, "You two are a swell team." We'd like to add that we think we *three* are a swell team.

Introduction to the Revised Second Edition

"Dr. Wasserman, I've tried to watch my diet, but it's all so compli-cated and technical that I've never been successful."

This was said by one particular patient of mine recovering from her recent heart attack. It was something I was hearing all too often. "It's too hard," "It's too complicated," "It's too much work," "Who can keep track of all that stuff," "I just need an easier way."

Then one day, a colleague hearing my lament introduced me to *Low-Fat Living for Real People*. He said, "My patients think it's great. Why don't you try using it?"

He was right. This **was** it! It made sense, it was easy to read and understand and it was fun. What cardiologist was the genius behind this book, I asked?

I was soon to learn the reason why this book was the answer. It wasn't written by a scientist or a physician, but by *real people*.

Linda Levy is a real person who experienced the family fear of heart disease, and Francine Grabowski is a nutritionist who deals with people struggling to understand low-fat living all the time. They were able to apply their real-life experiences and put to paper the answers to my patients' wishes.

This book is so entertaining it's hard to know you are learning while reading. But learning is what you do. What to buy, how to cook, how to snack and how to change your lifestyle. Most importantly, this book is about living and living well and longer. It's not about struggling or sacri-ficing or being unhappy. Try it, you'll like it; my patients certainly do.

Now if I can get them to write a version for my mother—*Low-Fat Living for Kosher People*—it would be a perfect world.

— Alan G. Wasserman, M.D.
Director, Division of Cardiology
Professor and Acting Chairman
Department of Medicine, The George Washington
University Medical Center, Washington, D.C.

Foreword(s)

S ince *Low-Fat Living for Real People* was first published, Francine Grabowski, my co-author, and I have visited dozens of cities and spoken to hundreds of people, all of whom are proud to call themselves "real people."

What makes them real people? They have to make dinner every night, whether they want to or not; they don't want to give up their favorite foods; and they are afraid low-fat food won't taste good.

Let me say that my husband, who is on a low-fat diet for medical reasons, absolutely loves good food. He has continued to eat this way for more than a decade because the food is delicious. And I still cook low fat because it is so fast and easy.

When we first began the low-fat life, we found the available books to be overwhelmingly technical, not to mention totally lacking in humor. *Low-Fat Living for Real People* is the book I wished I'd had all those years ago.

Let's go back in time.

Take a family whose favorite dinner was fried chicken and buttery mashed potatoes, whose idea of a great bedtime snack was ice cream (preferably vanilla fudge) with potato chips on the side, who thought the good life had something to do with thin-crust pizza with extra cheese.

In other words, take our family.

My husband and I have three children, the oldest two of whom were already away at college when the New Regime went into effect and we changed our eating habits. (The youngest refers to himself as "a foot soldier in the war against fat.") We had a reason for making the change.

It was a memorable day in March 1987 when the doctor said that my husband, who had experienced some discomfort in his chest, would have to have his heart "looked at." My husband pretty much wears his heart on his sleeve, but apparently that wasn't good enough – nor were the so-called "noninvasive" procedures (elaborate x-rays, stress tests, et cetera) that followed.

We couldn't imagine that anything could be wrong. Years ago this man had learned to confine his cigarette smoking, never very heavy in the first place, to the golf course. (If he were a golf pro, that wouldn't have been much help, but he isn't.) Although his job certainly falls into the sedentary category, he is very active otherwise, has never been over-weight, and has never had a cholesterol reading in the bell-ringing range.

No, we couldn't imagine that anything might be wrong. But *we* were wrong. Cardiac catheterization, a hospital procedure that allows doctors to see the heart from the inside, revealed some blockage in one of the main heart vessels, and so angioplasty was performed. (This is just like catheterization, except that a tiny balloon is inserted into a blocked vessel and is inflated and pushed through the vessel to clear away the fatty deposits.)

We learned from the cardiologist that many individuals in the United States over the age of forty have blocked arteries, which can lead to a heart attack. Sometimes you don't know how these things are going until it's too late. We felt lucky to have had a warning.

We learned, too, that studies are showing the problem begins early in life. Autopsies on the bodies of once-vigorous young people have revealed fatty deposits already forming in the heart vessels, a terrifying thought.

The good news is that changes in the way we eat can actually improve our chances of living a long and healthy life. Sounded good to us, and gave new meaning to the phrase, "The way to a man's heart is through his stomach."

Having cooked for a long time, I had my special recipes. In fact, when I heard that a friend was putting her favorite recipes on the computer, I resisted the urge to ask if she would henceforth be doing her cooking in the family room, where the computer is located. And I realized that my cookbooks and I had a system of our own; my favorite recipes were spat-tered with a number of their key ingredients, which served to wrinkle the pages so that I could open right to a particular recipe whenever I wanted to. At least as efficient as a computer.

I must say modestly that I am a good cook. Still, having established certain patterns over a quarter of a century, it was not easy to make many of the changes that were necessary. In fact, as I look back on it, I was in what I have come to call a "culinary depression" for about four months, months when I experimented with new recipes in an effort to make healthy dishes. I spent hours in the supermarket reading labels so that I could locate acceptable (from the standpoint of fat content) products. And I was afraid the food I cooked would be terrible. Well, the food I cooked *was* terrible. I followed recipes of the cook-your-way-to-a-healthier-heart type that said things like "Slice an eggplant. Broil until golden. Enjoy!" (Okay, okay, I made this up, but you get the idea. "Enjoy" we didn't.)

As I gradually became accustomed to cooking edible yet healthy foods, I met Francine Grabowski, a registered dietitian who helped us to "eat smart" – and collaborated with me on this book. We found that we share a basic philosophy, one summed up by the old saying: "Give a man a fish, you feed him for a day. Teach a man to fish, you feed him for a lifetime." Aside from our mutual concern about the woman who appears nowhere in this saying, probably because she is at home cooking the fish in question, we realized that books giving rules are the equivalent of giving a fish. This book is a fishing lesson.

It took a long time, but the happy day came when I realized I could cook food that was not only healthy and edible, but also absolutely delicious and very, very easy to prepare. Together, my husband and I learned to read labels and to ask appropriate questions when ordering in restaurants. With three other couples, we formed a gourmet club for healthy eating, meeting at each others' houses for potluck suppers that didn't involve cream sauces and thick cheese toppings. They, like us, were beginning to try to eat in a way that didn't scream "1950!" The eight of us became a support group, called ourselves "Ate is Enough," and had shirts made with the logo

"Ate is Enough" support group

◄

we designed: a cheeseburger with a line through it. The group continues to this day.

And so to *Low-Fat Living for Real People*. There are currently on the market all kinds of books about all kinds of problems for all kinds of diets. These diets deal with sugar, with salt/sodium, and so on. (Your doctor may have recommendations concerning your own particular diet.) But just about everyone seems to be dealing with the issue of lowering fat, and that's what this book is all about.

It is for you, whether you have had a problem already (fear is the great motivator), or whether you can simply read the handwriting on the wall. It will spare you a lot of what we went through in learning to adapt to a new lifestyle, and in learning to cook wonderful, quick-to-fix dishes. It will show you how to get your family on your side, how to eat out, but most important, how to live in this world. And I do mean live.

This is serious business, but it doesn't have to be depressing.

– Linda Levy

As a dietitian, I have coached people through life-saving nutrition changes related to preventing or even reversing the damage of heart disease, preventing the development of certain types of cancer, or decreasing the risks of diabetes. I have worked with people to set up the right conditions for success and cheered them on through countless days of practicing, stumbling, learning new skills. The "real winners" have gained the confidence and made choices to take control of their health.

More often than not, this nutrition coaching occurs at a time of crisis (whoever said necessity is the mother of invention must have been a dietitian). During my years at Deborah Hospital, a leading heart hospital in New Jersey, I became keenly aware of the fear, disbelief and overwhelming stress caused by the crisis of disease, not only for the patients themselves but also for their families. My work at Deborah fine-tuned my coaching skills: knowing the best nutritional techniques to help each person; tapping great reservoirs of courage in difficult situations; and helping to create realistic strategies for successful lifestyle changes.

I know what you are thinking…"I can't do this, it takes too much time to plan new meals or experiment with a new lower-fat version of a favorite food, much less learn new recipes." And then there's the taste bud issue (taste buds become pretty comfortable with the same old, same old and need retraining, too). Coaching for "real people" takes into account that most of us have on-the-go lifestyles, that change is difficult, and that a set of rules can take away from the pleasures of eating.

This book is about realistic changes for "real people," an "I can do it" approach, to move forward with humor and courage. Not coincidentally, I hear people who have made changes say, "I feel so good," "I have so much energy," "my family loves this recipe."

You may also be thinking, "nutrition information is too confusing." There *is* confusion about even the most basic information. To the dismay of dietitians everywhere, information about the good foods like vegetables, fruits and starchy beans can't compete with the advertising budgets of McDonald's, Coca-Cola, and Kellogg's. But there is an easy way to get sound advice – ask the experts. Registered Dietitians, who have had years of special training in nutrition, are uniquely qualified to help you end the confusion.

There are also times when a dietitian/coach works with a person who has committed the time and energy to learning about low fat, who knows that nutrition is a critical step in managing serious medical problems and who has created a joyful style of low-fat living. This is how it was when I met Linda Levy. Truly a leader, inspiring family and friends, taking every suggestion and making it better, her energy is contagious and inspirational. You'll see for yourself as you read this book.

Low-Fat Living for Real People is more than just information. It's an "I can do it" book, which is creative and fun, but most of all it is for your health.

– Francine Grabowski, M.S., R.D.

Chapter One
Leaving the Fat Behind

Leaving

the Fat

Behind

▲

*Cholesterol
is found
only in
animal
products
(meats,
poultry,
fish, eggs,
cheese and
other dairy
products).*

Getting the Facts Straight

First, a word from our sponsor:

Cholesterol

Yes, we, the food-buying public, are being sponsored by cholesterol. For years we have seen it everywhere, *everywhere*, particularly in its most popular form, "NO CHOLESTEROL."

Whoever thought that one up must still be laughing. Why? Because people are attracted to packaged foods that say "no cholesterol" thinking surely they must be healthier, but they probably aren't. So when cookies brag that they don't contain any cholesterol, well, that's because they have been made without animal products, but they still contain a lot of fat.

This whole business is further complicated by the fact that it's all too easy to confuse cholesterol in your *diet* and cholesterol in your *blood* ("serum"), which are not the same thing. If your doctor has ever taken a look at your lab results and said, "We're going to have to do something about this cholesterol," that was serum cholesterol he or she was referring to. (Speaking of doctors, any dietary changes made for a medical condition will need a doctor's supervision, so form a partnership with your doctor! This book is not a substitute for professional care.)

Because there appears to be a powerful link between high serum (blood) cholesterol and heart disease,[1] people are trying to lower cholesterol, and there is a great deal of information out there on how to do it: Eat plenty of fiber, raise the "good" cholesterol through exercise, and so on and on and on. Yes, there is information, much of it dry, some of it confusing, and not what you'd call eminently readable.

The fact of the matter is that serum cholesterol is only partly under your control (your body manufactures two-thirds of the cholesterol in your blood). Let's talk about one thing we *can* control: food.

♦   ♦   ♦   ♦

It's natural to assume that limiting cholesterol-rich foods in your diet will lead, automatically and inevitably, to lower cholesterol in your blood, and will improve the health of your heart. Sad to say, you could fill many a grocery cart with cholesterol-free foods, but these same foods could still be very high in fat. In fact, according to Jane Brody of *The New York Times*, considered by more than a few people to be the patron saint of health and fitness, "Far more important than the cholesterol eaten are the total amounts and kinds of fat in the diet."[2] In other words, restricting fat is the thing to focus on when you want to eat more healthfully. After all, we named this book *Low-FAT Living for Real People*, and it wasn't just because "low-cholesterol living" wouldn't fit on the book cover.

Why a low-fat diet? Because it has many health benefits, not the least of which is that it helps prevent clogged arteries,[3] and may also decrease the risk of developing diabetes and certain kinds of cancers.[4] In addition, a low-fat diet that focuses on fruits, vegetables, and low-fat dairy products is one that tends to lower blood pressure.[5] A nice bonus is that a diet low in fat (and, of course, calories) will result in weight loss.

A diet low in fat will also be low in cholesterol. (Organ meats – brains, liver, kidneys – are the exception and should be avoided. They are low in fat but high in cholesterol.)

Okay, so we're getting the idea that cholesterol is not the only villain in all this. But how to proceed?

By reading labels.

A diet low in fat will also be low in cholesterol, unless you are eating a lot of organ meats – brains, liver, kidneys.

Leaving

the Fat

Behind

Getting Organized

Reading labels is definitely the first step in getting organized, because labels will guide you through the miles of supermarket aisles and help you decide what foods to buy (or not to buy). The labels look complicated, but don't despair. Do the best you can for the moment, and by the time you come to the chapter that explains just how to use these labels to select low-fat foods, you'll find that *Low-Fat Living for Real People* has given you the necessary background to do that. You will be able to sift through and interpret the label information, and make it work for you.

Label Reading

Granted, that labels are destined never to make the best-seller list, and they are boring, boring, boring, but there's no getting around it: that's where the information is to be found. Unfortunately, labels are not made for easy reading, and, for those of us growing more farsighted by the millisecond, it seems as though they are printed in letters the size of a pinhead inscription of the Lord's Prayer. It would be a whole lot easier if crackers, for instance, came in a laundry detergent-sized box that could accommodate labels with VERY LARGE PRINT.

But they don't. So even if it means putting on your reading glasses in order to see labels clearly, it makes sense to read them if you're trying to eat less fat. You'll soon be convinced to buy differently, since many of the old standbys will be out-of-bounds. Take the time to check out the products that you buy routinely, such as crackers, cereals, cookies, and so on, and you'll be amazed to see the fat lurking there. Simply because a food is light, crisp, and non-greasy, you might assume that it is low in fat. You could, we're sorry to say, be mistaken, because fat may be precisely the ingredient that is providing the crispness.

The fringe benefits of label reading are enormous. Because you'll feel less and less inclined to buy some of the items you've been buying for years, you'll discover that there are long stretches of aisles in the supermarket you can avoid, thus dramatically cutting down on your shopping time. While the initial visits will take longer as you establish new buying habits, that won't last, and soon enough you'll be back on automatic pilot, mindlessly throwing groceries into the cart the way Mary Tyler Moore did every week at the beginning of one or another of her television shows while the titles ran. The only difference will be that you'll be throwing different things into the cart than you used to, and certainly different things than Mary Tyler Moore did.

The Pyramid

Remember the Four Food Groups (sounds like they might have had a hit single in the fifties)? They have been replaced by the Food Pyramid, introduced to Americans as a model for healthy eating, and useful also as a handy guide to foods that are low in fat. In fact, the Food Pyramid is the newest and best time-saver of them all.

Why a time-saver? Because it can help you decide quickly and easily which foods to buy. Then, as you stand in line at the check-out counter, pretending you're not looking at the tabloid headlines, you'll be confident that you've filled your cart with "all the right stuff."

You will save not only time but brain power if you simply fill your shopping cart with starches, fruits, and vegetables (all low in fat); the Food Pyramid honors all of these by placing them at or near the broad base. By contrast, put little in your cart in the way of fats, oils, and sweets, which you'll find perched in the tiny section at the top of the Pyramid.

As for the milk and meat level, the fat content is, unfortunately, not so clear-

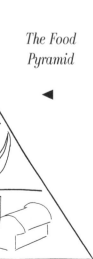

*The Food
Pyramid*

◀

cut. For instance, you'll see beans with meats, since both are high in protein. But unlike meats, beans are low in fat and high in starch. They coexist happily with the other starches at the base of the Pyramid and can be eaten in the greatest quantities.

So how do we know what to do with meats and dairy products? Never fear. *Low-Fat Living for Real People* will help you a bit later in this book.

Think of the Pyramid recommendations as relative. Plan to eat, for example, more pasta than meat. If there is a Food Pyramid drawn on the box of your favorite cereal, consider cutting it out and putting it on the refrigerator as a handy reference (Hint: wait until the box is empty before cutting).

The Wonderful World of Grocery Shopping

This is a very, very good time in the history of the Wonderful World of Grocery Shopping to be leaving the fat behind. You'll want to fill your shopping cart with foods that are pleasing in their taste and texture, foods whose colors are so appealing that they look wonderfully inviting on the plate. Variety is not only the spice of life, it is actually the basis for a healthy diet. Fortunately, it is a simple matter to increase the variety of foods you consume, now that supermarkets have grown to such a size that some of them deserve to have their own zip codes. They are stocked with all sorts of surprises.

Bell peppers, for instance, are now available in more than just traditional Christmas colors. Yellow, orange, and even deep purple ones can be found. Tropical and out-of-season fruits and vegetables are also commonplace these days. Besides the mushrooms that look like the little drawings in children's stories, there are others: shiitake (tiny parasols), huge Portobello (beach umbrellas), enoki (large toothpicks with tiny hats), to name a few.

Frozen vegetables have gone far beyond peas and carrots to include such items as asparagus, artichoke hearts, and snow peas. There's renewed interest in beans, and those cans, which once sat on the grocer's shelf gathering dust, today are being snapped up. Beans, both canned and dried, come in a wide variety: kidney, pinto, lentil, split pea (green and yellow), black-eyed pea, chickpea (alias garbanzo or ceci), Great Northern, navy, black, pink (rosetta), and even a bean called simply "small white bean." Ethnic foods are readily available – bean sprouts, water chestnuts, flour tortillas.

We've come a long way from bread shelves stocked primarily with the soft white stuff that some people think of as "raw," others think of as "the bread that doesn't spoil," and still others think of as "the bread you can play with." Bakery sections now feature all sorts of freshly made loaves, from white to whole grain.

Other aisles offer fresh as well as dried pastas, all of which come in shapes and sizes to suit your every mood. Vinegars have gone beyond red, white, and apple cider, and are flavored with herbs and fruits. Mustards are made in all sorts of interesting varieties, so you don't have to choose between the old standbys, the brown one and the bright yellow one that you find at sports stadiums and that make you want to break into a chorus of "Take Me Out to the Ball Game." The new mustards have names like "coarse and sassy" and may be made with wine, dill, honey, or champagne.

Tomato products, formerly pretty much limited to ketchup and tomato paste and canned tomatoes, today include crushed plum tomatoes with basil, recipe-ready diced tomatoes, pasta sauces, and the increasingly popular salsa (which just means "sauce" in Spanish, but where's the fun in calling it that?). Yogurts can be found that are fat free; some have fruit added, which may or may not be pre-mixed. One man we know was eating his first Dannon apricot yogurt, unaware that it required stirring, and was wondering why in the world it was called "apricot." "And then," he reported, "I hit gold!"

*Be adventurous
in the
supermarket:*

*Try a new
fruit.*

*Try a new
vegetable.*

CHAPTER

Leaving

the Fat

Behind

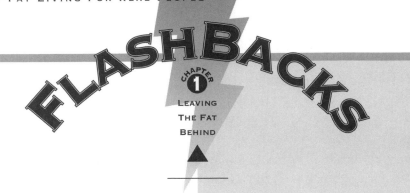

FLASHBACKS appear at the end of each chapter and are reminders of the key points in that chapter. (They should look familiar, and if they don't, you may want to go over the chapter again.) If you don't remember one other thing about *Low-Fat Living for Real People*, including who wrote it, please, please, PLEASE remember the **FLASHBACKS**. We'll start you off with a short list:

☞   End confusion: **choose fat-free or low-fat products.**

☞   **Eat plenty of starches, fruits, and vegetables.**

Chapter Two
Jack Sprat's Favorites

Jack

Sprat's

Favorites

*J*ack Sprat could eat **low** fat,
His wife could eat no lean.
And so betwixt them both, you see,
He outlived her by a long shot.

–Nursery Rhyme, updated

Best Bets: Starches

I t's fine to talk generally about food and recent advances in food, but what, you might well ask, are good choices? Which leads us neatly to the subject of STARCHES.

It may be, in an age when everyone talks about "complex carbo-hydrates," that when you think of starch, you think of laundry and ironing, but in fact starches are complex carbohydrates and this is as good a time as any to bring the word back into vogue.

There are people who already feel comfortable with starches, who nat-urally steer clear of fat-laden foods. They eat a vegetarian diet, lean toward organic produce, have an herb garden and a compost heap – and are not buying this book.

At the other extreme are people whose food choices are quite different, who believe that potato chips contain all the essential nutrients, who think that brown eggs are somehow healthier than white ones, who get their exercise by lying on the couch and watching workout videos, and who wish this whole thing about eating less fat would simply go away, the way that business about converting to the metric system did. (Although it didn't go away entirely. We'll be dealing with grams and milligrams on the food labels, and you can't get much more metric than that.)

Most likely you fall somewhere in between the two extremes, getting kind of anxious about this low-fat business, but not quite sure how to go about making what seem like earth-shattering changes in lifestyle. You will be delighted and relieved to see that many of the foods you recog-

Jack

Sprat's

Favorites

nize and already buy are actually good for you.

Chances are these foods are starches, and what makes them "good" is that they are very low in fat or fat free, and are therefore low in guilt or guilt free as well. Life can be beautiful.

So what is it that makes starches (the edible parts of plants: wheat, corn, rye, barley, rice, potatoes) so attractive? They contain fiber, vitamins, and minerals. By the way, you should know that all plants contain a tiny bit of naturally occurring fat, but this fat does not contribute to heart disease. On the other hand, some starches contain added fat, which makes them less desirable.

◆　　◆　　◆　　◆

B ecause starches are about to become your new best friend, let's take a look at them from the standpoint of stocking your kitchen cabinet. After all, if your shelves are loaded with fatty foods, that's what you'll eat. On the other hand, if those are starches in the cupboard, you'll be well on your way to better eating before you've even opened your mouth. Chances are you'll be eating more starches than you did before, and that's good.

(There is, however, the little matter of activity level. You can't expect to eat enormous amounts of anything, including pasta, without getting rounder and rounder, if you spend your days sitting at a desk and your evenings and weekends lying on a couch. Think about it. Human beings have an incredible ability to expand, and an expanding human being is more prone to heart disease. One man we know refers to his rotund condition as "enlarged skin.")

Think again of the Pyramid introduced in chapter one. You'll remember that it can help you make healthy choices – "all the right stuff" – quickly and easily. What follows is a pyramid of one particular type of food: starches. Again, the bottom of the pyramid contains foods that may be

"When did I get rounder and rounder?"

Jack

Sprat's

Favorites

eaten in the greatest quantity, in this case starches that contain no added fat. That is, you will not find any fat in the list of ingredients. At the top portion of the pyramid, starches do contain some fat. As a single food, eaten in a reasonable quantity, they present no problem. Still, if you are trying to limit the amount of fat you are eating, everything counts, so while you're at it, you might as well go with the no-fat-added starches in the bottom of the Pyramid of Starches.

The Pyramid of Starches*

Low-Fat
CRACKERS
(melba, saltine,
graham)

RICE (brown, white,
wild); **GRAINS** (barley, couscous, bulgar wheat, air-popped
popcorn); **BEANS** (dried, canned):
kidney, lima, lentil, split pea, navy,
chickpea, etc.; **PASTA** (formerly "spaghetti"); **POTATOES** (white, sweet); **BREADS**;
BAGELS; fat-free **CRACKERS** (including matzo);
fat-free **CEREALS** (hot, including oatmeal, grits,
cream of wheat, oat bran; cold, including corn flakes,
puffed cereals, bran); **PRETZELS** (fresh-baked soft pretzels;
fat-free pretzels); **CHIPS** (baked, fat-free only!); **STARCHY**
VEGETABLES (corn, peas, acorn and butternut squashes)

*There are other foods made with starches–specifically, fat-free bakery prod-
ucts–that have not been included in the Pyramid of Starches because they do
not offer the nutritional benefits of starches found here. Even though these
foods contain flour (starch), they also contain a lot of sugar, and while sugar
is "fat free," so to speak, and provides quick energy, it is without the health
benefits of starches. In addition, eating sugary foods reduces the likelihood
that you'll eat "good" foods – fruits, vegetables, and the kinds of starches
that appear in the Pyramid of Starches. To find out more about sugar in the
foods you eat, check the Endnote.[6]

Note that this is not an exhaustive list. Not to mention the fact that new products are coming into supermarkets every day. *Careful label reading, particularly the Ingredient List, will tell you specifically what products to buy and will guide you in choosing starches that contain no added fat.*

TO CHECK LABELS FOR SODIUM:

If sodium's something you specifically have to watch out for, check labels and choose:

"Low sodium" (140 mg or less per serving)
"Very low sodium" (35 mg or less per serving)
"Sodium free" (less than 5 mg per serving)

Obviously, the more you eat of a food that contains even a small amount of fat, the more fat you get. Because of fat content, serving size becomes a key issue in the upper section of the Pyramid of Starches. (If you're in the "I-can't-believe-I'm-getting-rounder-and-rounder" category, serving size is a key issue in general. You have two choices: Move more or eat less.)

Own Personal Serving Size (OPSS)

When manufacturers give information about fat, calories, and so on in their products, they use "serving size" as the reference point. This is fine now that most food labels are based on a serving of food that a person might actually eat. Still, *the serving size on the label may not bear any resemblance to the amount you, personally, eat.* Check the label to see what is considered the serving size, and then match it with your Own Personal Serving Size (OPSS). The next time you pour yourself a bowl of breakfast cereal, for instance, measure what you normally eat. If it's two cups, fine. That means the serving size of your cereal is two cups. But what if the box says the serving size is half a cup? Well, now you are eating *four times* the serving size on the label.

The serving size on the label may not bear any resemblance to the amount you, personally, eat.

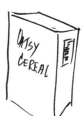

Jack

Sprat's

Favorites

*The label
law has
defined "low
fat" as 3
grams or
less per
serving.*

Let's suppose the label says there are 3 grams of fat per serving. The label will often say that, too, because the label law has defined "low fat" as 3 grams or less per serving.[7]

You have to do a little math to see how much fat you are actually getting in your two cups of cereal. Since your OPSS is four times that which appears on the box, you have to multiply the fat by four to find out that you have – all together now – 12 grams of fat per serving. Surprised?

If "grams" are unfamiliar, don't worry. A gram is simply a unit of weight, about that of a straight pin, and 28 grams are equivalent to something you are familiar with: one ounce.

So we see that it's not enough just to go with foods that say they contain no more than 3 grams of fat per serving, because your serving size might be considerably bigger than the one listed on the label, in which case those grams of fat are adding up faster than video game points.

One fine day (in our dreams) starches will edge out meats as the centerpiece of the American diet. What this will mean is that, if you serve dinner on the kind of sectioned plate once used for "Blue Plate Specials," the largest section will contain not meat, but starches, perhaps pasta or potatoes or a rice dish, and the meat (or chicken or fish) will go into a smaller section. In fact, you'll be able to answer the infamous question "What's for dinner?" without automatically mentioning first the meat, or chicken, or fish. It's the new, improved, Blue Plate Special. (Once again--If you're in the "I-can't-believe-I'm-getting-rounder-and-rounder" category, remember: The size of the new, improved Blue Plate is no bigger than the old one.)

Beans, the All-Star Starch

On some level, we have known for a long time that beans are good for us. There was even a childhood rhyme about beans being good for the heart, a rhyme we were not allowed to say in front of grown-ups. (If you'd like a refresher lesson, turn to the Endnote[8] for the

**Starchy
Beans**
*black
black-eyed peas
cannellini
chickpeas
fava
Great Northern
kidney
lentils
lima
navy
pink
pinto
split peas
white beans
whole peas*

prime time version.) The undesirable side effect, namely, flatulence, or gas, will be less of a problem as your system becomes accustomed to eating beans.[9] A few drops of a product called "Beano" (available in pharmacies), when added to the first forkful of beans that you eat, may also help.

Beans really are good for us. Why? Fiber, fiber, fiber.[10] STARCHY BEANS (dried or canned) are low in fat, too. In fact, you'll see them right there in the big, lower section of the Pyramid of Starches (see page 28).

Beans come in a wide variety of colors, shapes and sizes, and can be used in many dishes. Canned beans are the easiest to use. Drain and rinse them well (they'll be less gooey and salty) and throw them into just about any soup – vegetable, chicken, whatever – or toss them with your salad. Or you can open the can of beans a day ahead and put the rinsed, drained beans in a bowl with some fat-free bottled dressing, then let the whole thing marinate in the refrigerator until you toss that salad. Or add the beans to frozen, mixed vegetables (thawed but uncooked), and marinate together (see recipe for Marinated Beans and Vegetables, page 185).

Dried beans are fine, too, but they require pre-soaking plus a couple of hours or so to cook. You can soak them overnight in cold water, or you can boil them for two minutes and then let them sit (covered) for one hour. In any case, discard the soaking water and add fresh before cooking according to package directions.

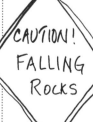

Be aware that you might possibly find a little rock or two in the package along with the dried beans. These have to be removed, because, unlike beans, they will not soften no matter how long they are cooked. When we say that beans contain minerals, this isn't what we have in mind.

Beans offer a pleasant change of pace. One day when you find yourself in the supermarket idly wondering when they'll invent a new meat, try beans. Beans are in the mainstream now; you'll even see them on the

Jack

Sprat's

Favorites

Fruits
apples
apricots
bananas
blackberries
blueberries
cantaloupe
cherries
dates
figs
grapefruit
grapes
*honeydew
melon*
*mandarin
orange
sections*
mangos
nectarines
oranges
papayas
peaches
pears
persimmons
pineapples
plums
prunes
raisins
raspberries
strawberries
tangerines
watermelon

menu in nonvegetarian restaurants. Recipes are all over the place, too. You'll find them on the bags and cans in which the beans are sold, as well as in cookbooks and newspapers and magazines – and in the back of this book, for that matter. Just make sure your recipe uses no more than one teaspoon of fat per serving. You may be surprised by how much you like beans.

Best Bets: Fruits and Vegetables

There are other complex carbohydrates that contain virtually no fat but do contain plenty of vitamins and minerals, the old standbys, as well as other amazing goodies, some as yet unidentified. As a package – that is, as food – they are essential to a healthy heart, and may indeed protect it from disease.[11] These complex carbohydrates are the ever-popular FRUITS AND VEGETABLES. When we studied nutrition ("Health") with Miss Miller back in sixth grade (she wore her hair in a bun, didn't believe in lipstick, and made sure her long, gray cardigan sweater was buttoned up to her neck), fruits and vegetables were one of the basic food groups, and they're still around. Unlike some other food groups we could mention, they have never fallen out of favor. Remember Carmen Miranda with her hat loaded with fruit? Turns out it was a low-fat hat.

While fruits and vegetables retain their celebrity status – we should be eating five servings a day – not everyone actually eats them. *Moby Dick* remains a great book, but does everybody read it?

Consider fruit. *More than half of all adults* don't eat even one serving of fruit a day.[12] Sobering, when you consider that not much in the way of preparation time is needed to peel a banana, let alone simply bite into an apple (as Adam found out, to his dismay). They are the ultimate easy-access fruits. The original fast food.

As for vegetables, more people eat them, but what they mostly eat are potatoes, and the potatoes are french fries and potato chips.[13] Not too impressive, is it?

Of course preparation of vegetables is required, which isn't exactly enticing. They have to be peeled, sliced, diced, chopped, minced, or grated. Food processors can help, unless left untouched in the kitchen cabinet. If used, they have to be dismantled, washed, and then reassembled, all of which can be off-putting for people who don't get much more high tech than the little gadget that removes apple cores. But there is another way to get your vegetables, one which you may find more–ahem–palatable. Think "salad."

Salad Shortcuts

Eating salad is, of course, a great way to get your vegetable quotient for the day, and there is a tool-free approach to its preparation, one that doesn't even involve a knife or cutting board. In the supermarket you can buy everything you need, already cut up and ready to go. You'll find tiny little carrots, peeled and washed (keep them in a bowl of water in the refrigerator, so they'll be juicy instead of dried out); shredded cabbage; cute little pieces of broccoli, ditto cauliflower; sliced mushrooms; bite-sized cherry tomatoes. You will even find washed, packaged lettuce leaves of all kinds.

Or you can spin your own lettuce with a salad spinner. Yes, it's more time-consuming than using already-washed lettuce that you buy in the market, so what are the advantages of doing the washing? Taste, primarily. And appearance, since the deep green leaves are greener, the pale green are softer. They are crisp and springy, tender and delicate, sweet and nutty and tangy. Tossed together they produce a "burst of flavor." Talk about a taste sensation!

A salad spinner is both a wildly useful tool and a boon to people who used to let their lettuce dry on towels spread all over the kitchen – and dining room, too, if lots of company was coming.

As long as you are spinning lettuce, remember that iceberg lettuce is almost entirely devoid of nutrients. You have only to remember the Titanic to know that icebergs don't have what you'd call an enviable reputation, so you might want to think about selecting another, darker green

CHAPTER 2

Jack

Sprat's

Favorites

Vegetables
artichokes
asparagus
beans
broccoli
Brussels
sprouts
cabbage
carrots
cauliflower
celery
cucumbers
eggplant
greens:
   beet
   chard
   collard
   dandelion
   kale
   mustard
   turnip
leeks
mushrooms
okra
spinach
sprouts
squash
zucchini

Jack

Sprat's

Favorites

(and therefore better for you) lettuce, such as romaine. Romaine will keep for several days in the refrigerator if it has been washed, spun, and bagged in plastic. You could also use spinach, bibb lettuce, or another leafy green, or even a combination of these. You might even add those marinated beans mentioned earlier, throw the whole thing together, and make one spectacular, prize-winning salad.

That prize might even be a spouse! We were standing in line at a buffet dinner and overheard someone exclaim, "I want to marry the person who made that salad!"

Other Shortcuts

Frozen vegetables require no washing at all, just opening a box or tearing open a bag (Scissors? Knife? Teeth?), making it easier than ever to eat vegetables with all their heart-protecting qualities.

Introduce yourself to some starches, fruits, and vegetables.

▶

There are those that come in upscale, foil-wrapped boxes, "frozen vegetables for the rich and famous" – vegetables such as asparagus spears and whole green beans picked at their peak. Gently cooked in the microwave, they may be mistaken for fresh. If you think of ordinary frozen vegetables as being a product of the supermarket, think of these as a product of the vegetable garden. Imagine a vegetable garden with no weeding necessary! Even if you've never been too crazy about frozen vegetables, you might want to try them.

Frozen vegetables (or a combination of frozen and fresh) can be added to leftover pasta or rice. Sort of "Leftover Helper." If you've ever dreamed of being an Arctic explorer, try it out here, in the freezer section. You might even find something you wouldn't come across in the produce aisle – like artichoke hearts. You never know.

Canned vegetables are another possibility, but they may well be mushy, bland, and/or salty. Still, they are better than no vegetables at all. (It's seven o'clock. Do you know where your can opener is?) They can be heated, dumped into soup, or used as weights in an aerobics class.

But what if you don't like vegetables, have never liked vegetables, have absolutely no interest in eating vegetables? For your heart's sake, consider that they have come a long way from the days when they were a soggy, beige side dish. As we've just seen, without even being cooked, they can be put in salads. Lightly cooked and tossed with chicken or fish, they add flavor, color, and texture. Fully cooked and puréed, they can be used as a sauce. Overcooked, they can be thrown out.

Still unconvinced? Well, if you only eat your vegetables with a cheese or a mushroom soup sauce, you've never really tasted vegetables. (And you're adding a lot of fat.)

You can roast 'em

You can toast 'em

You can tell your friends and boast 'em.

You can steam 'em

While you're dreamin',

You can simmer

(And get slimmer)

You can grill

And get your fill.

You can sauté, you can bubble,

'Cause it isn't any trouble,

You can cook 'em every way,

Just eat your veggies EVERY DAY!

Jack

Sprat's

Favorites

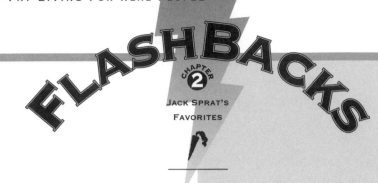

☞ **Best Bet:** Buy starches with no added fat. Always check the Ingredient List.

☞ **In the running:** Buy starches with a little added fat. Make sure there are no more than 3 grams of fat per serving. More than that is too much.

☞ **Try BEANS!** Versatile, delicious, and easy to use, they are the All-Star Starch.

☞ **Create a new, improved "Blue Plate Special"** that features grains, beans, or pasta in the largest section of the plate.

☞ **Pay close attention to your OPSS** (Own Personal Serving Size). The bigger your OPSS, the more fat you may be getting. You may also be getting rounder and rounder.

☞ **Other Best Bets:** Buy (and eat) fruits and vegetables. Count your blessings – salad counts as a vegetable!

Chapter Three Protein Reconsidered

Protein
Reconsidered

Center Stage No More: Meat and Poultry

Meat and poultry have customarily occupied a privileged place on the dinner table, the main event at the main meal of the day. When we remember the Sunday roasts of our childhood, we conjure up a scene that Norman Rockwell would have been crazy about. We remember a heavily laden dinner table with bowls of mashed potatoes, boats of gravy, baskets of buttered biscuits. We remember quantity, going back for seconds and maybe even thirds. We remember good food, good times, good feelings, with an occasional squabble over who would get the end cut.

Back when a "roast" referred only to food, not to a bunch of individuals making wisecracks about some "honoree," people loved eating it. But why put it in the past tense? There are a lot of families out there who still love it, who know the best way to make sure the kids come home for dinner is to announce that a roast will be served. Even older, married kids can often be lured back this way. Beans and rice just don't hold the same fascination.

The taste of a roast, like anything else, is acquired, and the fact is that you've simply gotten used to eating it, lots of it, maybe. Possibly you have weekly barbecues where you roast something enormous on a spit in your backyard.

Or it may be that you have cut down on your meat eating. After all, these aren't the first words you've read on the subject of reducing fat in your diet, and you might well have gotten wind of the fact that meat is where a lot of the fat is. So let's say you're eating less meat, and that you're making do with a life-sized, full-color cardboard cutout of a medium-rare roast beef in the middle of the table in lieu of the real thing.

When people are eating less meat, they're often eating chicken instead, low in fat yet comfortably familiar. You're probably already doing that, and you can feel confident you are moving in the right direction. (This assumes, by the way, that you are not eating chicken *wings*, which are, unlike other parts of chicken, high in fat.)

If you're on a real poultry binge, chances are good that you are eating so much chicken you have come to the point where you say things like "If I see another piece of chicken, I'll grow feathers." That's a sure sign you have fallen headlong into the dreaded chicken rut, and are tired of building your meals around chicken. The best way to climb out of the chicken rut, without going back to mashed potatoes, gravy, buttered biscuits, and roast beef, is to introduce yourself to some starches, fruits, and vegetables that you might have overlooked in the supermarket. The "embarrassingly simple recipes" at the back of this book will help you.

We must be clear on this: We are not saying you should give up meat. Or chicken, for that matter. We are saying you might want to take another look at them – how often you eat them, and how much you eat at one time.

A Little Goes a Long Way

Cutting down on the amount of meat and poultry you eat will, at the same time, reduce the amount of fat you consume, including Mr. Big of the Fats World, SATURATED. It all comes down to the fact that *cutting down on your serving size is the most important of all dietary changes*. Yet people balk at doing this. Maybe they have old myths ringing in their ears, something about needing lots and lots of protein. But in fact you need to eat only small amounts of meat or poultry, because you don't need much protein each day.[14]

News *Flash*:

Your protein does not need to come from an animal or a fowl. It might come from beans, and it might come from whole grains and vegetables, too. Studies show that there tends to be less heart disease among people who eat vegetarian diets.[15] (There are different types of vegetarian diets, the strictest of which does not include anything that comes from animals. Keep in mind that a great many vegetarian recipes include ani-

Cutting down on your serving size is the most important of all dietary changes.

CHAPTER
3

Protein
Reconsidered

*The serving
size for
meat and
poultry is
3 ounces,
something
like a deck
of playing
cards.*

mal by-products like eggs, cream, butter, and cheese, which makes them very high in fat. You can bet these are not the kinds of recipes that were used in the studies just mentioned.)

We aren't suggesting you become a vegetarian, only that you be aware that non-animal protein offers two advantages: ❶ You don't need to think about the serving size of chicken or beef or whatever; and ❷ you don't need to worry about fat. Take heart. Literally. You can do it. (See chapter 10, "Foods Your Heart Will Love.")

Let's get back to serving size, because the fact is that most of us are used to eating meat or poultry every day. We've discussed serving size earlier (OPSS – Own Personal Serving Size), but it warrants more discussion here.

If you've ever been to a steak house, you've been introduced to outlandish portions that have absolutely nothing to do with what we're talking about here. A restaurant that serves meals whose centerpiece is 16 or more ounces of cow flesh really should be located near a heart hospital. Besides, a steak like this has to be served on an incredibly large plate – let's face it, a platter. Shouldn't you be able to fit your food onto a normal-sized dinner plate? If you find yourself eating from serving platters, you might want to rethink portion size.

Yessiree, a 16-ounce serving is outlandish, but it may be even more outlandish than you realize. The recommended serving size for meat and poultry is – you'd better be lying down for this – *3 ounces, something like a deck of playing cards*. No one is proposing that you share that 16-ounce steak with three friends (and even at that, you'd get more than 3 ounces), but the idea is to begin to cut down on serving size, which will cut down on fat, including saturated fat. Then, too, as you cut down on the amount of meat and poultry you eat, you will naturally eat more starches, vegetables, and fruits, which is the whole idea.

(Also, as you cut down on these serving sizes, you'll be cutting down on cholesterol, since – we've said it before and we'll say it again – a diet low in saturated fat will also be low in cholesterol, unless you are eating a lot of organ meats.)

When you cook your own meat, you may have heard that you should

Protein

Reconsidered

"allow for shrinkage," which is to say that the meat weighs more before it's cooked than after. That's true, but you can't buy a slab of meat the size of a Kleenex box and expect the cooked weight to be appropriate. To put it in perspective, if you buy a pound of lean ground beef, by the time you allow for shrinkage during cooking (25 percent), that pound of beef will make four heart-healthy, low-fat living hamburgers of about 3 ounces each.

That's LEAN Meat We're Talking About

If you're eating meat, what to buy? It's not which animal you eat, but what part of the animal. You want lean, not fatty. This goes for poultry, too. (By the way, most of the fat in chicken and turkey is housed neatly in the skin, so by dispensing with it, you are that much ahead. If you look underneath the skin, you'll also find a few unappealing little hunks of pale yellow fat, which should be removed before cooking the chicken.)

Up to this point in our discussion, we have talked about "low fat." But now we're talking about meat and poultry, and The Powers That Be instead use the terms "Extra Lean" and "Lean." Extra Lean has half the fat and saturated fat of Lean, and you don't have to bother going to butcher school, because you'll know the meat or poultry is acceptable *provided you eat only 3 ounces*.

Even if your meat department isn't using Extra Lean and Lean stickers, you can still get nutrition information, since the label law requires that it be readily available. However, the information might be anywhere – on the meat, on the counter, posted on the wall – or it might be scribbled on sheets of paper stuck underneath a cash register someplace, in which case you'll have to ring the bell and ask someone for the information you need. Just in case your meat department doesn't have readily available information, or if the "meat in question" doesn't say "Extra Lean" or "Lean," you can fall back on the old method of consulting a list of cuts of meat that qualify. (Note that these are "extra lean" only if you eat no more than three ounces. The more you eat, the more fat you'll get.)

Buy "Extra Lean" or "Lean" meat.

Protein

Reconsidered

"EXTRA LEAN" CUTS OF MEAT

No more than 5g of fat (2g saturated) in 3 ounces

BEEF: Eye round, tenderloin
GAME: Venison
PORK: Cured ham (butt end)
POULTRY: SKINLESS Chicken breast, turkey breast

"LEAN" CUTS OF MEAT

No more than 10g of fat (4.5g saturated) in 3 ounces

BEEF: Flank steak (fat trimmed), top round, bottom round, rump
PORK: Canned ham (shank end), fresh lean ham
POULTRY (SKINLESS): Dark meat of turkey and chicken (*Except chicken wings! Very high in fat!*)

Ground beef is, unfortunately, something else altogether. The USDA (Department of Agriculture), which is responsible for labeling meats, hasn't gotten to ground beef, so hamburger doesn't follow the same rules. What this means to you is that you'll find no consistency from one store to another as to what is called "Lean." (Chances are you won't find any ground beef labeled "Extra Lean.") The terms "percent fat" and "percent lean" are thrown around until your head spins. So – until things are clarified on the ground beef front, pay no attention to claims on the package that this is "Lean," because it may or may not be. Instead, rely on Nutrition Facts, and remember the real definition of "Lean": contains no more than 10 grams of fat per serving and 4.5 grams of saturated fat.

And what if there are no Nutrition Facts on the package, which there may very well not be? You'll just have to ask the butcher. Annoying, isn't it?

As for lunch meats, they often say "97% fat free" (or 96% or 98%). Sounds good, but this is very, very misleading, making you think the product is low in fat even if it isn't. Sometimes the manufacturers add a lot of water during processing.

If they would take out the water (fat chance!) from a lunch meat that calls itself "97% fat free" and then show you the fat content, you'd see that the lunch meat may be as much as 50 percent fat, not 97 percent fat free at all. A good choice? We don't think so!

The fact is that certain lunch meats share only the vaguest family history with cows and pigs and chickens, which makes you wonder why they are called "meats" in the first place. They come packaged in perfect squares and circles and have names like "bologna" and "olive loaf." When was the last time you took your child to a petting zoo to see an olive loaf? Don't buy lunch meats and assume you are buying meat.

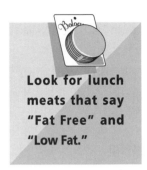

Look for lunch meats that say "Fat Free" and "Low Fat."

Best Bet: Fish

Fish is a different, well, a different kettle of fish. It contains protein, all right, but fat is not an issue, even if you've heard some fish rcfcrrcd to as fatty. (Besides, there's very little saturated fat in any fish.) There are people who don't eat salmon and mackerel, for example, because they are fatty fish, but the truth is, *all fish are appropriate for a heart-healthy diet*. In fact, eating fish may very well be the easiest way to reduce the risk of heart disease.[16] Only if a fish is deep fried or otherwise cooked in a lot of fat is it the kind of "fatty" you'll want to avoid.

Naturally, if you eat a variety of fish, you'll get a variety of benefits. You don't have to eat large amounts of fish, either. Just two meals a week, with a serving size of 3 ounces at each meal, will do the trick, an amount that will be, by now, a familiar quantity.

As for shellfish, which is very low in fat,[17] suffice it to say that it has an undeserved reputation for raising serum cholesterol. Enjoy it occasionally; there is no reason to avoid it, unless, of course, you are keeping kosher.

The recommendation to eat fish more frequently is really nothing new. But maybe you harbor a lingering resentment because of all those Fridays when you had to eat fish. Or maybe you think it smells bad (comedian Elayne Boosler asks, "How do you know when herring has

"How do you know when herring has gone bad? Does it smell good?"
– Elayne Boosler

gone bad? Does it smell good?"), but we assure you, fresh fish doesn't have an unpleasant odor. Then, too, when you think "fish," maybe you immediately think "fresh fish," which makes you think of making yet another shopping trip, which in turn makes you throw your hands up in dismay and opt for a nap.

That extra shopping trip has to do, of course, with the fact that fish spoils easily and you can't just keep it around, although if yours spoils overnight, your refrigerator may not be as cold as it should be. Fish will keep longer if you put the package in a bowl filled with ice cubes before putting it in the refrigerator.

So if you can't keep fresh fish on hand, how about frozen? There's no question that it loses a lot in the translation, which is to say a lot of the taste goes in the freezing process, but it is certainly better than no fish at all. Frozen fish sticks, however, bear about as much resemblance to fish as ginger ale does to champagne, so don't go eating frozen fish sticks and think you're eating fish. Maybe when you were a kid you drank ginger ale and pretended it was champagne, but you probably don't want to eat fish sticks and pretend they're fish. Besides, chances are the breading has a lot of fat in it, the very thing you're trying to avoid. Check the label.

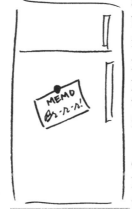

But there is another alternative to fresh fish, and that is canned, yes, canned, convenient and easy to keep on hand. Needs no refrigeration, either. All right, so you're having a little trouble envisioning a long, flat can with a flounder inside. You may even be wondering why you never noticed it in the supermarket, an impressive can like that, somewhere near the tuna. We admit we've never seen canned flounder either, but to be perfectly honest, when we mentioned canned fish, we were thinking (besides tuna) of salmon. Some canned salmon has the extra added attraction of bones, and although you may doubt that anyone on this earth would want to pick out bones, we hasten to add that that's precisely the point: you don't pick out the bones. You shouldn't pick out the bones. They fall apart easily as you mash up the salmon and you'll never notice them, but they'll be there nevertheless, providing you with a nice source of calcium. A simple way

Is your refrigerator cold enough?

to use salmon is by making a tuna salad using salmon instead (see recipe for Crunchy Tuna Salad, page 181), and if you want to feed a lot of people, you can buy salmon in a can big enough to be mistaken for soup. (If there's a center bone in that big can, we suggest you remove it, rather like you take out the center plug from a fresh pineapple prepared by that exotic machine in the supermarket.)

Proceed With Caution: Cheese

People get their protein from meat, from poultry, from fish and shellfish. They also get their protein from dairy products in the form of milk, cottage cheese, yogurt, and cheese. Like all dairy products, cheese is an excellent source of calcium and protein but it is also an excellent source of fat.[18] Now, because we are a nation of cheese-lovers-who-are-trying-to-lower-their-fat-intake, cheese manufacturers have been playing around with low-fat, even no-fat, cheeses. They've had a few minor problems with the stuff, like getting it to melt. You might ask yourself just what it is you're dealing with. One woman put some leftover broccoli on a baked potato, topped it with fat-free cheese, and popped it into the microwave. When she took it out, the cheese was nowhere in sight. She found it later, when she'd finished eating the potato and broccoli. There it was, stuck fast to the plate.

We've had similar problems ourselves. One that comes immediately to mind was a failed attempt at making a fat-free grilled cheese sandwich in the toaster oven. Suffice it to say that a putty knife had to be called in to scrape the congealed cheese off the rack, sides, and window of the toaster oven.

As for the taste of the fat-free cheeses we've met–ohboyohboyohboy. You might as well send your taste buds on vacation. The cheeses are soapy, and some of them are so rubbery they actually bounce. (Don't ask how we happen to know this, but trust us. They bounce. Toys "Я" Us

Protein Reconsidered

Protein
Reconsidered

**1 ounce
cheese =
1/4 cup
grated
cheese**

probably has a cheese aisle.) Still, even though the flavors and textures are nothing like the original, if you are of the persuasion that a day without cheese, not orange juice, is like a day without sunshine, then by all means go for it.

In fact, there is a low-fat cheese (no more than 3 grams of fat per ounce) that has been around for a long time – long before people were talking about how much fat there was in cheese. Although it doesn't have the familiar ring of cheddar, mozzarella, and Swiss, it has the advantage of being untouched by modern technology. The name of this cheese is sapsago; you might want to try it. It is a hard cheese, so you'll grate it. (It has a lot of flavor *and* a strong odor, so be forewarned.) You could also stay with old-fashioned cheese, the kind mother used to buy, and just use less of it. In fact, an ounce of cheese, which doesn't look like much, actually comes out to be 1/4 cup of grated cheese, enough to lightly cover an entire casserole. But if you can already picture yourself scraping off the entire cheese layer and putting it on your own plate, you'd do well to consider eliminating cheese from your day-to-day diet. This doesn't mean that you'll never have another pizza. It simply means that cheese moves away from the everyday and into the realm of "occasional treat."

Variety, Variety, Variety: A Typical Week

Now that you know you can eat meat, poultry, fish and shellfish, and cheese, the only thing left to do is to eat all of them. Over the course of a week, though, not all at once. And in 3-ounce servings, too. Remember the old adage, or something close to it: "Variety is the seasoning of existence."

Since different foods offer different benefits, plan a week's meals that include a variety of foods. Instead of serving chicken four or five nights out of seven, try the following pattern: chicken or turkey, two nights; fish or shellfish, two nights; vegetarian, two nights; one night, your choice. We chose leftover turkey, but you might choose beef or pork. Add a salad or hot vegetable and some fruit, and you have a complete, delicious, low-fat meal. Make it simple. Embarrassingly simple. And delicious. Like these recipes, which are designed to see you through a typical week.

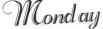

Monday
Shrimp with Tomatoes (see recipe, page 207) and rice

Tuesday
Grilled Turkey Breast (see recipe, page 199) and baked potato

Wednesday
"Mexican" Eggplant (see recipe, page 171)

Thursday
Rice, Pasta, and Spinach (see recipe, page 144)
with leftover Grilled Turkey Breast (see recipe, page 199)

Friday
Carefree Flounder (see recipe, page 202)
and Embarrassingly Simple Rice (see recipe, page 150)

Saturday
Bean and Pasta Soup (see recipe, page 174)
and Veggie Burger (buy frozen)

Sunday
All-Purpose Chicken (see recipe, page 195)
and Not-Too-Boring Potato-Onion Casserole
(see recipe, page 146)

Protein
Reconsidered

Retro Living:
Back to Balanced Meals

L et's remember that we're talking not just about food but about meals, which are nothing more or less than foods in combination. The phrase "a well-balanced meal" echoes all the way back to our childhoods – with good reason, it turns out. First of all, we used to sit down to eat that "well-balanced meal" all together, as families. Today, we often can't eat together, what with everybody's busy schedules, but the truth is, we often don't even sit down to eat. Not a great habit to stand at the refrigerator with the door flung open, picking your way through dinner, eating a "meal" that is far from balanced.

Balance is important, and that, too, goes back to childhood. You'll recall being on the playground, playing on a see-saw, and you might also remember what happened when your friend suddenly decided to get off and go over to the slide while you were still hanging in the air. Down you came with a crash and your best friend suddenly wasn't.

When you eat a "good meal," which is to say a well-balanced one, you give your body a smooth ride, and that is good for your heart. Nothing jarring. No unexpected bumps. You do that by picking from each level of the Pyramid (heaviest on starches, fruits, and vegetables). Then you eat your meals with some regularity, maybe every five or six hours, and you have a smart snack in between (see chapter 6) if you're really hungry.

Keep your heart happy. A simple thing like eating complete meals can reduce your risk for heart disease.[19]

How much, what, and when you eat, all affect your risk of getting heart disease.

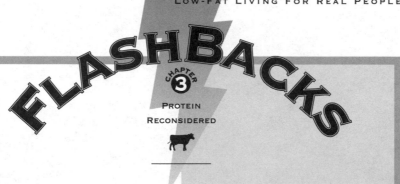

CHAPTER **3**

PROTEIN
RECONSIDERED

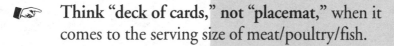

☞ **Think "deck of cards," not "placemat," when it** comes to the serving size of meat/poultry/fish.

☞ **Choose "Extra Lean" and "Lean" meats.**

☞ **If you eat lunch meats:** Choose those that say "fat free" or "low fat."

☞ **Take a break from chicken every night.** Make fish, beans, or vegetables center stage.

☞ **Eat complete, well-balanced meals for your heart's** sake.

Chapter Four

Ms. Sprat's Favorites

Ms.

Sprat's

Favorites

Worst Bet: Saturated Fat

It isn't very hard to know what's what in the Fats World. Saturated fat is about the worst of the dietary offenders, the fat most closely associated with heart disease. A "killer fat," you might say. Doesn't sound all that great, does it? You've seen it rear its ugly little head in the meat/poultry/cheese combine, but it lurks menacingly in many other places as well: butter, cream, sour cream, cream cheese, ice cream, and other high-fat dairy products. The good stuff, in other words. This means that not only do we have to change the way we eat, we also have to change the rhymes we teach our kids: "I scream, you scream, we all scream for – fat-free frozen yogurt!"

Better Bet: Monounsaturated Fat

*Olive and
canola oils
are "better
bets."*

Saturated fat is not the only fat; it is simply, as we've said, the worst offender. However, you must consider all kinds of fats, since TOTAL FAT is the issue here. Maybe we should coin a word and simply call all other fats "faturated." Let's examine them.

Apparently the best bet, from the point of view of heart health, is monounsaturated, of which olive oil and canola oil are prime examples (as are avocados and nuts). Those who live in Mediterranean countries have known the secret of monounsaturated fats for a long time, use olive oil in their cooking, and have a very low rate of heart disease. (Bear in mind they also eat plenty of starches, fruits, and vegetables, and there's a good chance they walk to the market every day.) Canola oil doesn't have the history of olive oil, but it may well have the promise.

What do we mean when we say that monounsaturated fats are the best fats for heart health? What would you say to less chance of heart attacks? Less chance of death from heart disease?[20]

If you are confused about what fat to use in cooking, you may want to go with these oils, but go easy: no more than one teaspoon added fat per serving. Nobody is recommending that you deep fry your pasta in monounsaturated oils.

> ### SPEAKING OF OLIVE OIL, A QUICK DIGRESSION.
>
> You might logically think that, if olive oil is a fat of choice, olives would be a good thing to eat. After all, where does olive oil come from? As a matter of fact, one of the writers of this book is a devoted olive fan. (We won't talk about the other.) But because olives are a fat, even though a particularly "good" fat (monounsaturated), you'll want to think of them as garnishes, not main or side dishes, and use them accordingly, to enhance the taste and texture of other foods. The same is true for avocados and nuts, whose oils are also monounsaturated.

And Then There's . . . Polyunsaturated Fat

Besides monounsaturated fat, there is the famous polyunsaturated fat, very commonly used but losing its "good guy" status. Although it first appeared that polyunsaturates were innocuous even in large quantities, that now seems not to be the case.

What are some examples of polyunsaturated fat? Most of the oils that you use in daily food preparation are polyunsaturated. Some of these are: safflower, sunflower, corn, sesame, cottonseed, and soy. But you don't have to memorize long lists. You already know that olive and canola oils are monounsaturated – read "good." Fats of animal origin are saturated (as are tropical oils such as coconut, used less often in processing foods today than they used to be) – read "bad." Everything else is polyunsaturated.

Ms.

Sprat's

Favorites

A CAUTIONARY TALE:

On top of everything, there is another kind of fat, *trans* fat, that may mimic the effect of saturated fat on the body. Found in (hard to spell much less pronounce) HYDROGENATED and PARTIALLY HYDRO-GENATED FAT, it may well turn out to be as harmful as saturated fat.

Ah, the wonders of modern science! A chemical process known as hydrogenation takes a poor, unsuspecting vegetable oil and changes it so that it becomes solid and spreadable (margarine, shortening), and lengthens the shelf life of the products it is found in (such as crackers and bread). Food labels won't help you spot *trans* fat, because, as of this writing, specific information on *trans* fat has no place on the label. But foods containing hydrogenated or partially hydrogenated fat will say so on the Ingredient List.

And there are many such foods. Besides being found in lots and lots and lots of the packaged foods you buy (chips, crackers, cookies, and other commercially baked goods), hydrogenated fat is commonly found in margarine.

People are actually proud of the fact that they use margarine instead of butter, brag about it to their friends, use it as a sign of how they've solved the problem of using too much fat (as far as fat content is concerned, margarine, like butter, is all fat[21]), and therefore how they're protecting themselves against heart disease. They see margarine as a reasonable alternative to butter, but the truth is, if hydrogenated fat is in there, it may not be.[22]

The newer margarines that contain no hydrogenated or partially hydrogenated fat – *trans* fat – are an obvious improvement over butter, as are diet margarines, which contain less fat. Both, however, leave a lot to be desired when it comes to taste.

A far better alternative is jam or jelly, which contains no fat at all, but is, admittedly, not very useful for sautéing.

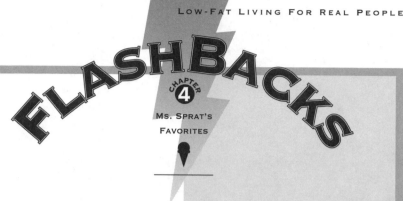

☞ **Remember** that saturated fat would be voted Least Admired by members of the Academy of Fats if there were such a thing. It is found in meat, in poultry, in cheese and other dairy products, and earns a definite "thumbs down."

☞ **Best Bets:** Use monounsaturated fats, such as olive and canola oils.

☞ **Best Bets II:** Because they are monounsaturated fats, use avocados, nuts, and olives. Hint: use only as garnishes.

☞ **While you're at it, remember** that both hydrogenated and partially hydrogenated fat may be saturated fat copycats as far as the body is concerned. They are found in margarine, chips, cookies, crackers, and commercially baked goods, and also earn "thumbs down."

Chapter Five
Sizing Up Fat

Understanding Quantities

Now that we know what kinds of fats are out there, let's talk about quantities, because we need to have some understanding of how much fat we are taking in, and how little we should be taking in, to help keep ourselves healthy.

FOOD WE MAKE: Normally when we cook our food, we measure in teaspoons, tablespoons, and cups. We like teaspoons.

FOOD WE BUY: It's too bad that, when we shop for food, we are forced to think in the language of labels, that is, in GRAMS. We remind you that a gram is a very, very small unit of weight (there are 28 grams in an ounce), about that of a straight pin. What do grams have to do with teaspoons?

HOW MANY TEASPOONS IN A...		
1 tablespoon	=	3 teaspoons
1/4 cup	=	12 teaspoons (4 tablespoons)
1/2 cup	=	24 teaspoons (8 tablespoons)

There are 5 grams of fat in a level teaspoon, whether oil or margarine or any other fat, unless it is one of the new, lower-fat versions. (All cooking oils contain the same amount of fat, so don't be misled by special blends and the like.)

TEASPOONS INTO GRAMS		
1 teaspoon oil	=	5 grams
1 tablespoon oil	=	15 grams
1/4 cup oil	=	60 grams
1/2 cup oil	=	120 grams
1 cup oil	=	240 grams

Here is an easy-to-use conversion chart, showing how much fat (in grams) is found in common household measures.

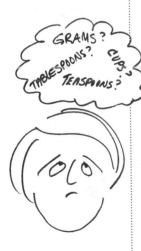

Measuring in Grams, Courtesy of "The King"

You may or may not be happy to hear that Elvis Presley has come back from the dead (assuming you believe he's dead) to help us understand how to think in both kinds of measures, that is, teaspoons/tablespoons/cups on the one hand, and GRAMS on the other. When we think of Elvis, we think of his hit song "Are You Lonesome

Tonight?" which asks the musical question, "Is your heart filled with pain?" It's an excellent question indeed when you consider that Elvis reportedly had a fondness for red-eye gravy, which is almost entirely bacon grease. In fact, the drippings from one pound of cooked bacon (just to keep measurements simple), mixed with a little black coffee, makes enough red-eye gravy to pour over biscuits and serve four. Hazardously. (Hey, kids! Don't try this at home!)

We'll give Elvis's mother, Gladys, one thing: her recipe was undoubtedly embarrassingly simple. But if she had measured the drippings when she cooked that pound of old-fashioned, fatty bacon, she would

---

> ### "ARE YOU FAMISHED TONIGHT?"
>
> (To the tune of "Are You Lonesome Tonight?")
>
> *Are you famished tonight?*
> *Are you famished tonight?*
> *Are you sorry you can't eat much fat?*
> *Does your memory stray*
> *To your porterhouse days*
> *When your steak was the size of a mat?*
>
> *Does your vegetable platter*
> *Seem overly bland?*
> *Do your beans, rice, and pasta*
> *Seem overly planned?*
>
> *Is your heart filled with pain?*
> *(Not if you're eating grain!)*
> *Tell me, dear, are you famished tonight?*

---

have found there was just over a cupful, or 260 grams of fat from the whole pound of bacon, which means that one serving has *sixty-five grams of fat* (260 divided by 4). M-m-m-m BAD.

We bid a fond farewell to the "ignorance is bliss" era of the fifties and return to the present, when we are (or should be) concerned about the amount of fat we take in each day.

Spreading the Fat Around
A Daily Diary

Why worry about teaspoons, tablespoons, cups, or the 65 grams of fat in red-eye gravy? Because we're leading up to the idea that there's a limit to how much fat is appropriate to take in each day – on your bread, on your salad, in your cooking. The Big Picture.

Sizing

Up

Fat

In order to better understand the notion of quantity, we need to look again at margarine, a very commonly used, yet much misunderstood, form of fat.

How much margarine might you use in a normal day? It makes sense to see how it slips in, since it tends to be overused, creeping into the diet without being recognized as a contributor toward total fats.

Maybe you put:

1 teaspoon on hot oatmeal

1 teaspoon on a piece of toast

2 teaspoons on a sandwich at lunchtime

1 tablespoon on green beans at dinner

2 tablespoons in mashed potatoes, also at dinner

If you had spent the day measuring and counting, you'd see how much fat you had consumed in the form of margarine: 13 teaspoons, more than half a stick, in a single day. This does not account for additional fat you've ingested in salad dressing or mayonnaise, in cookies, crackers, or other snacks. It doesn't account for any fat you might have used in cooking a chicken breast, for example, let alone the fat found in the chicken breast itself. It doesn't leave room for any monounsaturated fats, such as olive or canola oil, which might actually have some health benefits. And yet those 13 teaspoons are the equivalent of 65 grams, something like a serving of that deadly red-eye gravy mentioned above. (If you are partial to math problems, check the Endnote[23] to see how this was worked out.) Fat adds up very, very quickly.

Using Fat in Recipes

Another example of the use of margarine can be found in baking. We've selected oatmeal cookies because they sound so wholesome. This genuine, bona fide recipe yields 48 cookies. It calls for:

2 1/2 cups oats	1 cup brown sugar
1 3/4 cups flour	1 teaspoon baking soda
2 eggs	1 teaspoon vanilla
1/2 cup granulated sugar	1/2 teaspoon salt

1 CUP MARGARINE

We'll spare you the blending and the beating and the adding and the mixing and the dropping-by-teaspoonsful-on-greased-cookie-sheets. The bottom line is that our batch of cookies contains 1 cup (48 teaspoons) of margarine, or one teaspoon per cookie (5 grams). If they aren't burned, it wouldn't be hard to polish off 13 cookies, a baker's dozen, but look how much fat they contain: a grand total of 65 grams.

Putting It All Together

Remember Elvis's red-eye gravy? And the bits of margarine at meal times that added up to half a stick? And the 13 home-made oatmeal cookies? They have something in common, which is that they all contain about 65 grams of fat. You're not going to forget this number, because you'll see it on food labels everywhere. Here's why.

Believe it or not, there are researchers who have devoted their lives to figuring out The Big Picture, the limit to how much fat should be consumed each day, and 65 grams is the number they came up with, the number you'll see on those food labels. This may not exactly be your personal number, which depends on size and activity level, but it's in the ballpark. (If you want more information on determining your personal "fat limit," there are many, many texts available on the subject.[24])

Sixty-five grams, then, is a number that you need to be familiar with. It is MORE THAN ENOUGH FAT FOR AN ENTIRE DAY on a relatively low-fat diet, according to the food label. As it is, Americans have so much fat in their food that it's amazing they don't just slide out of bed in the morning. There are people who actually get close to half their day's calories from fat. The thinking is that if fat could be reduced to no more than 30 percent of a day's calories, people would also reduce the likelihood that they'd fall prey to the evils of heart disease. (The figure "30 percent" gets a lot of press, and you may have heard it tossed around.)

But there's no need to get all involved with numbers. Stick with Jack Sprat, not Jack Sprat's wife, in the supermarket.

Stick with Jack Sprat, not Jack Sprat's wife, in the supermarket.

CHAPTER
5

Sizing

Up

Fat

FLASHBACKS

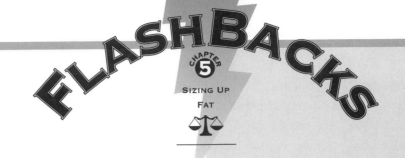

CHAPTER
5

SIZING UP

FAT

☛ Remember that there are *5 grams of fat in 1 tea-spoon of oil.*

☛ **Sixty-five grams of fat is more than enough for an entire day.** Spread it throughout the day, rather than taking it all in at once (a serving of red-eye gravy, 13 cookies, whatever).

Chapter Six
Snacking

The Mindless Event

SNACKING is a common way for fat to creep into the diet, because fat is found in all sorts of packaged foods, from cookies and cakes to chips and crackers. It's too bad, but snack foods as we know and love them are associated with high fat and pleasure and chips and chocolate and cheese and dips and nachos. (Think of "junk food" as the contradiction in terms that it is.) You can probably conjure up one or two occasions when these things didn't appeal to you, but you'll probably also recall that you were in bed with a stomach virus at the time.

Snacking itself is not necessarily a bad thing (depending, of course, on what you snack on). That is, the body is actually designed for small, frequent meals. However, the body is not, repeat not, designed for small, frequent meals plus one or two big meals every day, which is what a lot of us have.

The trouble is, snacking becomes a kind of mindless event, a way to get through some of the shows that miraculously find their way onto the television screen. The mindlessness means that you won't be thinking about fat content and serving size, certainly not about your OPSS (Own Personal Serving Size), and it doesn't take much to go from OPSS to OOPS! Let's use Wheat Thins as an example of doing just that. (We've chosen Wheat Thins because one of us was more or less addicted to them in a former, higher-fat, life.)

Say you sit down in front of the TV with a box of Wheat Thins and eat the whole box, and say you are compulsive enough that you counted them out as you were eating them. You'd know you just ate 160 crackers. Check that label and you'll see one serving is 16 crackers, but that your Own Personal Serving Size (OPSS) was, at least on this particular occasion, *ten times* that on the label.

How much fat are you getting? The label will tell you that there are 6 grams of fat per serving. Multiply that times your 10 servings, and you'll come to the unhappy realization that you've just consumed 60 grams of fat. (If you're in the "I-can't-believe-I'm-getting-rounder-and-rounder" category, the issue is not only that you've eaten all that fat, it's that you've eaten all *that*.)

How could you have stopped yourself from eating the whole box of crackers? We've had a certain amount of success closing up the box and flinging it across the room. Being too lazy to get up and go after it, we don't eat any more crackers. We've also found it useful to throw the uneaten crackers into the garbage and cover them with coffee grounds. Even our beloved Wheat Thins are not all that appetizing in such a condition.

The Addiction

Snacking is complicated and food manufacturers know that. So maybe they use a little fun and a little humor to divert you from the issues. Take SMARTFOOD Popcorn, for example.

Calling a food SMARTFOOD may be a clever marketing gimmick (since it is clearly not the food that is smart but the people who buy it), but we like to think that consumers aren't so naive as to judge a product by its name alone.

Or by its package. There is a pleasant cleverness about the messages on bags of SMARTFOOD Popcorn. At one time there were little testimonials, sent in by satisfied customers, printed on the back of the bag. One such testimonial, in the form of a poem, began, "I crave it every minute," and went on to confess an inability to resist eating SMART-FOOD popcorn. Snacking, the addiction.

Let's take a look at the Reduced Fat White Cheddar Cheese version. (Remember, "reduced fat" means there's at least 25% less fat in this version than in the original, but that still leaves a lot of fat.) According to the label, the bag contains five servings of about three cups each. We're here to tell you that there were 172 kernels in our three cups. How long does it take to eat those 172 kernels? Funny you should ask. It took one of us eight and a half minutes to consume them, working slowly and steadily,

CHAPTER
6

Snacking

*Typical
snack foods
have little
place in a
low-fat diet.*

eating three to four kernels at a time. We all know that people often tend to eat popcorn *quickly* and steadily, and they may not stop eating after eight and a half minutes. If you can't resist eating SMARTFOOD popcorn, if you just can't stay away from it, who knows? The whole bag may be your serving. There's even a message on the bag telling consumers that SMARTFOOD has reduced the fat content by 40% "so you can eat even more!"

But there is the small matter of OPSS. The label states that a 3-cup serving contains 6 grams of fat, so if you are addicted enough to eat the whole bag, all five servings just for you, that's 30 grams of fat. You might just as well sit down and eat a quarter of a stick of margarine. Yummy-yum? We don't think so.

Where does this leave us? The truth is that no matter how clever the label is, or what's on it, including "reduced fat," you'll get a lot if you eat a lot. And if you eat a lot, you'll get rounder and rounder.

Snacking for the Chocoholic And the Chipsoholic

We've been suggesting healthy snacks. But what if you want chocolate, crave chocolate, ABSOLUTELY HAVE TO HAVE CHOCOLATE? Add Hershey's syrup to fat-free milk and have a glass of fat-free chocolate milk. If this sounds too healthy, have a fat-free Fudgsicle, which will give you the flavor (but not the fat) of chocolate. Or make a sundae with fat-free frozen yogurt and that same Hershey's syrup.

If these fat-free versions of chocolate don't satisfy your cravings, stick to dark rather than milk chocolate. Cocoa butter (found in dark chocolate) appears to be less harmful than butterfat (found in milk chocolate). But you'll have to read labels to make sure the chocolate you are buying does not contain butterfat. Remember, too, that where fat is concerned, serving size becomes important. You can cut down on serving size by buying really expensive chocolate, because of course you'll buy less. You can cut down even further by sharing it with your very best friends.

And what if you crave potato chips, cannot imagine life without that fatty snack? First of all, there are the newer, baked versions. But there's no getting around it, these don't taste like high-fat chips. If that's what you are craving, then take an occasional fat holiday. Factor the chips into your diet, using your fat for the day in snack form. This will mean having no additional fat that day and making sure to eat plenty of starches, plenty of fresh fruits and vegetables, and putting a fat-free dressing on your salad in order to allow for fatty snacks.

You have to plan for this. If you are going out to eat, or if food will otherwise be out of your control one day, don't pick that day to consume your day's fat in potato chips. And, needless to say, you won't eat unlimited quantities of chips. You'll read the label, be shocked to see how much fat is in them, and then figure out what serving size will fit into The Big Picture of total daily fat. A 6-ounce bag of chips contains *60 grams of fat*, otherwise known as "enough fat for the entire day."

Plan, plan, plan.

The American Heart Association has come on board with this kind of thinking, and has issued reduced-guilt guidelines. The idea is to think in terms of several days, not day by day or meal by meal. While overall fat intake remains the same, if you indulge in one meal, simply be extra careful for the next few days. No big deal. Again, plan, plan, plan.

CHAPTER
6
Snacking

The Fat-Free Chocolate-Covered Creme-Filled Mini-Cakes Diet

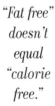

T he latest trend in snacking is getting the fat out, and we most certainly have the technology to do it. Liposuction, the popular surgical technique that sucks the fat out of thighs and other parts of the body where it is deemed undesirable, is now being used on food. Or something like liposuction, anyway. Food manufacturers, ever anxious to jump on a lucrative bandwagon, even if it's a health-oriented one, are flooding the market with fat-free versions of everything they can get their hands on.

What this means is that, if your sole focus is on lowering fat, watch out. You might very well find yourself on the *Fat-Free Chocolate-Covered Creme-Filled Mini-Cakes Diet*. If, as they say, "you are what you eat," you could be in trouble.

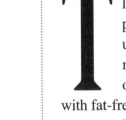

It's a fat-free diet all right. Fat free and sweet. Very seductive. If your aim is to lower fat, you might think that Fat-Free Chocolate-Covered Creme-Filled Mini-Cakes would be just the thing to have at breakfast. And again at lunch. And at snack time, too.

Oh, by the way, did we mention that the Fat-Free Chocolate-Covered Creme-Filled Mini-Cakes Diet is a weight-*gain* diet? That "fat free" doesn't equal "calorie free"? And that great minds are asking: No fiber, no fat, no vitamins, no minerals – what in the world is this?

If you have never eaten Fat-Free Chocolate-Covered Creme-Filled Mini-Cakes, you might want to know that not everyone falls in love with them. Plenty of people find that taking out the fat has made them chewy and hyper-sweet, with a lingering taste that even strong, black coffee doesn't wash away. Then again, if you want to have one piece of cake and taste it for the rest of the day, this could be for you.

One man, whose birthday cake was made from the stuff, blew out the candles, ate the first piece, and said, barely containing his disappointment, "Why didn't you just sing 'Birthday to You'?" Then the ice cream

"Fat free" doesn't equal "calorie free."

was served. Well, it wasn't exactly ice cream. It wasn't ice milk, either.
It was . . . it was . . . "frozen dessert."

Fat-Free Chocolate-Covered Creme-Filled Mini-Cakes are not the
answer to getting the fat out. Real food is vastly preferable, so look first
for starches with no added fat, look carefully at starches with added fat, and
look with suspicion at starches from which the fat has been liposuctioned.

Smart Snacking

Snacking

Someone could make a lot of money with a line of healthy snack
foods. They could be called "Sound Bites," a take-off on the
media term you hear all the time. Or maybe Good-4-U-Snax
–"Snack your way to a healthier you!" There they'd be, an array
of packages you could put on your shelf, open whenever you felt
like a snack, and know you were getting a nutritious low-fat or
fat-free snack that, not incidentally, tasted absolutely wonderful.
Trouble is, what you'd find when you opened up those Good-4-U-Snax
would be six fat-free saltines, an apple, and a glass of fat-free milk star-
ing up at you. Not exactly what you had in mind, is it?

Luckily, Chocolate-Covered Creme-Filled Mini-Cakes are not the only
snacks that have come on the market with "FAT FREE" in banner letters
across the package. There are others that, while not exactly "Good-4-U,"
come a lot closer than those Fat-Free Chocolate-Covered Creme-Filled
Mini-Cakes do. They are made from starches such as corn or rice or
potatoes (like baked potato chips), and become crispy snacks without the
addition of fat.

Sometimes, though, the words "FAT FREE" appear big and bold on the
package, but there is fat on the Ingredient List. How can this be? The
answer is simply that so little fat was used in processing that the product is
considered fat free. ("Fat free," according to the label law, means there is
less than half a gram of fat in one serving.) However, if the fat listed is
hydrogenated or partially hydrogenated, find another snack.

Still, if you want less fat in your diet and at the same time you want to
eat real food, you'll have to think about snacking the way you think about

*Avoid
snacks
containing
hydrogenated
fat.*

CHAPTER
6

Snacking

eating in general. Try filling up with something starchy (but if you find that filling up makes you rounder and rounder, don't fill up quite so much).

Go back and check out the Pyramid of Starches. You could have bread or sourdough pretzels (salted or unsalted depending on sodium restrictions, and check the label to be sure they are fat free), even a bowl of cereal with fat-free milk. Popcorn is a good choice, but make sure you air-pop it. Even microwave popcorn is – surprise, surprise! – high in fat, especially when you take your OPSS (Own Personal Serving Size) into account.

IF YOU WANT TO BE A LITTLE INVENTIVE

Try leftover new potatoes or corn on the cob. Fat-free crackers and chips go nicely with salsa or with bean dips. New products are coming on the market constantly, so keep your eyes open and see what's around. Starches have the enormous advantage of making you feel satisfied.

Smart Snacking: The Plan of Attack

In case you haven't noticed, snacking and socializing go hand in hand. You go to the movies, you snack. (Buttered popcorn? Shoebox-size box of Milk Duds?) You take a break at work, you snack, maybe hit the vending machines. (Peanut butter crackers? Potato chips?)

You can still snack and socialize; it's just that your snacks will be different. If you know where you spend your time, you can find out in advance where you can get low-fat snacks. In other words, know your territory. This thinking applies whether you are socializing or not. If you spend time in the mall, say, know where you can buy fat-free frozen yogurt, or a fancy coffee or tea. If you pass convenience stores each day, know which ones sell bagels and fresh fruit and fruit-flavored seltzer. (Seltzer? Yes, because if you feel hungry, you might really be thirsty! Strange but true, maybe, but a glass of water often takes care of "hunger.") If you're working in an office building, know what time the cafeteria opens so you don't have to rely on those vending machines.

We've said it before, we'll say it again: Real food is vastly preferable, so that's what to look for when you feel like snacking.

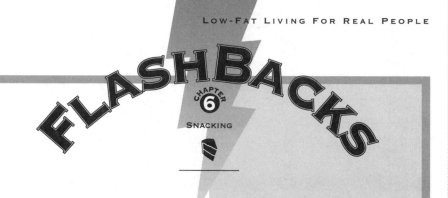

FLASHBACKS

CHAPTER **6**

SNACKING

☞ **Plan snacks carefully and SNACK SMART!**
Because snacking is a mindless event, you can take in a lot of fat very quickly. It doesn't take much to go from OPSS to OOPS!

☞ **Check out the Pyramid of Starches.**
Eat real food–starches–for snacks.

☞ **Good snack choices:**
Bagel, apple, banana, raw carrot
Fat-free crackers or chips with bean dip or salsa
Fat-free pretzels (unsalted, if you are trying to eat less salt)

☞ **If you crave chocolate:**
Try a fat-free Fudgsicle.
Try fat-free frozen yogurt with Hershey's syrup.

☞ The Fat-Free Chocolate-Covered-Creme-Filled-Mini-Cakes Diet sounds good but **isn't**, so –
Look first for starches with no added fat.
Look carefully at starches with added fat.
Look with suspicion at starches from which the fat has been "liposuctioned."

☞ "Fat free" isn't "calorie free."

Chapter Seven

Exercise: Moving Away from Fat

Exercise:

Moving Away

from Fat

Making A Case For Exercise[25]

If you eat too much food, even fat-free food, you'll find yourself getting rounder and rounder, the traditional reason for exercising. Traditional, but not only. Muscles work better when they are used, and the heart is a muscle, the "muscle of choice" in this case. When you get your blood flowing, you exercise your heart. (Before making changes in your activity level, you should, of course, check with your doctor.)

Like a lot of people, you may feel that "exercise" amounts to putting forth a major effort just in order to sweat, shower, and change your clothes in the middle of the day. It means stopping whatever you are doing, going to the gym (alias "health club") and "working out" surrounded by other people who are working out and apparently having a wonderful time (are they hired for this, or what?), their already-perfect bodies clad in merciless exercise outfits that offer no hiding places for unsightly bulges. Going to the gym means riding a bike that doesn't go anywhere, taking a long walk on a short treadmill, and climbing stairs that stay put.

Did Cave Man go out to exercise? Or, for that matter, Cave Woman? Well, yes, as a matter of fact, but they didn't call it that, and they certainly didn't go to a gym to do it. Exercise was built into their lives, since common, everyday activities, like grocery shopping, were pretty arduous back then. By contrast, our lives are often physically undemanding, and so we compartmentalize exercise, give it a special time of day, a special name, and buy special clothes to wear when we are doing it. But there is another way to stay (or become) physically fit, without resorting to exercise videos and health clubs and spandex.

Exercise: The "Fun" Part

In your search for The Ideal Exercise, keep in mind that you don't have to call it "exercise." In some circles, the term "physical activity" has come into vogue. Call it anything you like, as long as you are motivated to do it. And what will motivate you? Who knows? We met an elderly woman who told us she entered a 2-mile fun run. It seems the woman in front of *her* was wearing gold shoes, not your standard walking shoes. All we know is that she was not about to be beaten by a pair of gold shoes, and she beat the woman wearing them, as well as her own previous best time.

Remember: ❶ nontraditional forms of aerobic activity are fine; ❷ you have to do whatever it is regularly – three to four times a week should be about right; ❸ it's okay to enjoy yourself. Anything goes, as long as it keeps you moving vigorously for thirty minutes. You'll know you have selected the perfect activity for yourself when you don't realize the allotted time has passed.

Why nontraditional aerobic activity? Because the workout aspect is incidental to the pleasure of performing the activity. If you like doing something, you'll do it, and that's the key, not just talk about it, but do it, and do it regularly. (A friend of ours tells us that he runs "three miles *a time*." He may run regularly, but apparently he doesn't run often. Still, he's clever. We'll give him that.)

Say you love rowing a boat. Great! But how often can you do it? If you have ready access to a rowboat (not to mention water), you're all set. Or say you love conducting an orchestra. Also great! But if you can only occasionally get to a boat – or an orchestra – well, that brings up something we should discuss.

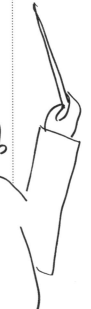

Exercise:

Moving Away

from Fat

Variety:
Also the Spice of Exercise

You can vary your activities. The easiest in terms of convenience, accessibility, and necessary equipment, is walking. So maybe you take a good, brisk walk in the early morning several times a week. But if you're bored, try other aerobic activities from time to time, like dancing. (Aerobic activity makes your heart beat faster, makes you breathe harder, makes you take in more oxygen.)

Dancing? Yes, dancing. It can be one of the great nontraditional aerobic workouts going. Dancing can be enjoyed alone or with a partner, and there are dances to suit almost everyone, whether young and tired or old and vigorous. Pick your style.

Unlike aerobics, the object of which is to finish (". . . five and four and three and two and one!"), the object of dance is to continue. There is whirling, gyrating, turning, bending, reaching, twisting, arms and legs moving continuously to music, and the music keeps you going, catches you up so you don't think about time, don't think about anything at all, hypnotized as you are by repetitive movements, you just keep going, you don't stop, no one stops, as long as the music is playing.

Now it just may be that you like going to a gym, that your personal "Stairway to Heaven" is a stair-climbing machine, and you don't think of it as a set of stairs that stays put. Maybe you like rowing, but you prefer a rowing machine to a boat on a lake. Maybe you'd rather do your cross-country skiing indoors, where it's warm, using a device built for exactly that. Of course that's fine, and you'll have plenty of company.

But if you hate the idea of working out, let alone changing your clothes to do so, then try something – anything! – else. Your body will love you for it.

Moving Every Day

Let's say you've just read the last section and you're thinking, "Yeah, yeah, yeah. You're not going to catch me doing anything like that!" Well, there is another way. Instead of a heavy-duty workout several times a week, you can go instead for a moderate workout every day. You'll want to do thirty minutes of activity, but here's the good news: it doesn't have to be all at once. For instance, maybe you want to walk briskly for only ten minutes, then rake leaves for ten minutes later in the day, then still later do some good, heavy housework. Ten, ten, ten: there's your thirty minutes, and it may have been easier to carve out of your day than a single thirty-minute chunk. The point here is that you must DELIBERATE-LY carve it out of your day, because with all the things you have to do, if you're not careful, exercise will make its way right down the list of priorities until it drops off altogether. You certainly don't want this to happen. It doesn't matter how you feel (as in "I just don't feel like exercising today"). What matters is how you *will* feel, how you'll function, and how you'll look, too. In other words, it's worth doing because of the enormous benefits your body will reap, both inside and out.

The fact is that many of us take better care of our cars (change the oil regularly, and so on) than we do of our bodies. True, this is an era of replaceable body parts, but let's face it; you go through life with one body and you want to take good care of it.

We've been talking about heart-health activity, but there's other activity you might call "just moving around." This is definitely something you want to do – move around. If you don't, one fine day you discover you really can't do it anymore. Everything is conspiring to keep you from moving around, because things have gotten too convenient. There are long-handled mops, brooms, dust pans and brushes so you don't have to bend over. Trash compactors mean you rarely have to take out the garbage. Leaf blowers equal "no raking," and snow blowers mean the same for shoveling.

Exercise:

Moving Away

from Fat

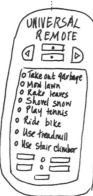

Convenience has gotten just a little out of hand. Think about the ever-popular universal remote control, designed for people who don't want to have to reach for other controls. They can just hold one and lie there. There's even a lamp that turns on and off with the sound of a clap instead of the old-fashioned "get up and walk over and turn the thing off."

We know people who have gotten so lazy we suspect they've arranged with the recycling gang to pick up their daily newspapers directly from the driveway, so they won't have to bother walking out to get them in the morning.

How to keep moving around? You may not have thought of it before, but inconvenience can actually help you do it.

If you keep things you need all the time OUT OF EASY REACH, you'll move more and feel better. Try putting what you use most often on an upper shelf, not one you need a ladder to reach, just one you need to stretch a little to reach. Or on a lower shelf, one that you need to bend down to reach. This applies to your favorite mug in the kitchen, sweatshirt in the closet, the toothpaste in the bathroom. Note: If you have a tendency to topple over, put things down low rather than up high.

Now – where did we get the idea of keeping frequently-used items on inconvenient shelves? From a woman named Rusty who happened to be sitting next to us on a plane. Moral: You never know where your next bit of useful information will come from, so listen up! The reverse is also true: You have some good information now. Pass it on!

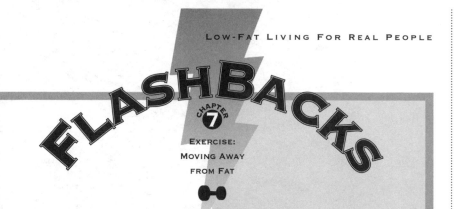

FLASHBACKS

CHAPTER **7**

EXERCISE:
MOVING AWAY
FROM FAT

☞ **It's okay to enjoy yourself.** If you choose the right exercise for yourself, you won't realize the allotted time has passed.

☞ **Exercise regularly**, about three to four times a week.

☞ **Sustain vigorous activity for about thirty minutes.**

☞ If you prefer, **do three 10-minute bursts of activity each day.** Think "10-10-10."

☞ **Carve out your exercise time** from your day.

Chapter Eight

Strategies for Eating Out

Eating in Restaurants: Replacing Fat Gram Counters with Common Sense

Actually there are two ways to eat out: in a restaurant and at someone's house. While the restaurant is more expensive, it's a lot easier to deal with, assuming that it's one where the food is carefully cooked to order. Unfortunately this is not true of "all you can eat" places, where everything is already prepared when you arrive, and they are just waiting to see how much you really can put away. Portions tend to be enormous, which translates into an unacceptable amount of fat.

When you eat out, it's hard to know just how much fat you're getting in your food. However, if you keep your fat intake under control the rest of the day, then, when you go to a restaurant, all you'll have to do is order sensibly, and you're about to see how to do that. You won't have to burden yourself with one of those fat gram counters you see everywhere, either. Instead of sitting there thumbing through a book, the way you do when you're visiting a foreign country where you don't speak the language, you'll be free to enjoy your meal – which is, after all, the whole point.

Restaurants: Out with Friends

Sometimes life has a way of working out. By the time you have concluded that Twinkies are not one of the basic food groups (well, not part of the Pyramid), you've reached the point where you no longer have to be one of the crowd, ordering what everyone else orders, never mind if their taste runs to foods so rich and heavy that you have to sign a medical release before you consume them. On the other hand, if you still want to have friends, it might be better not to point out their poor food choices just now. Soon enough your habits will begin to show, and you'll find that as they start in on an enormous slab of fatty roast beef, they'll say something like, "Boy, I haven't eaten meat in six months!" Better not mention that they said that last week, and the week before, too, come to think of it. Watching you eat may be making them feel guilty.

And they may become "friendly enemies," people who mean well when they urge you to eat something that won't hurt "just this once."

Just this once. Think about that for a minute. In theory, just this once wouldn't matter, of course. But in practice, it would be possible to have 365 unacceptable dishes per year (366 on leap year) and that could spell trouble. It could also make you rounder and rounder. Note that these foods may still crop up on special occasions, but that a "special occasion" involves more than merely going out for dinner. Think "Birthday with a Zero in It"; think "Major Anniversary"; think "Unbelievable Job Promotion."

IF YOU EAT AT RESTAURANTS FREQUENTLY, YOU CANNOT CONSIDER EVERY RESTAURANT MEAL A SPECIAL EVENT. It is merely a convenience, a chance to have a meal without the nuisance of preparing it. When delicious but fatty foods come your way, which they will routinely if you're eating in restaurants, you'll have to be strong about this: Stand pat, stand firm, stand up for your rights. This may come in the form of a gentle shake of the head (as in "No, thank you"), or a firm "No, thank you."

Tips on How to Order

Study the menu. Think "no cream, no cheese, no butter" (Sat Fat). Order foods that are broiled or grilled rather than fried, passing up things like deep fried fat, tempting though they may be, and popular, too, heaven knows. Avoid dishes that are described as "pan-fried," "crispy," "au gratin" (with cheese), "Parmesan" (with Parmesan cheese), and "scalloped" or "escalloped" (sounds like scallops are involved, but most often it is something that finds itself awash in a rich sauce).

Study the menu, part II. Think "mix and match," because you really can pick anything that's offered. Don't feel you're limited by the way the

Think:
no cream
no cheese
no butter

Strategies

for

Eating Out

restaurant has organized the dishes. For instance, you might see a fish dish that is served in a butter sauce, but maybe another dish comes with a fresh tomato and herb sauce. Clearly they're prepared to make both sauces, so all you have to do is ask for the tomato and herbs instead. Next, find the vegetable that most appeals to you, keeping in mind that it might be hidden in another dish completely ("served on a bed of asparagus"), choose the rice or potato you prefer, and add them to the entree of your choice. You'll wind up with a dinner that is the envy of everyone at your table.

Talk to the server, your link with the kitchen. You might consider saying that you are on a "medical diet." Since restaurants customarily consider it bad for business when a patron keels over during the main course, they will be much more likely to comply with your wishes.

You are about to make a number of demands, but at the same time, you don't want to appear to be demanding. One woman we know has gone to the extreme, and asks so gently and so quietly that hers is often the order that never finds its way to the kitchen. You can be more demanding than that. You have a right to be. It's your own health and well-being, and you can be cheerful but firm in requesting certain things.

Ask to have vegetables rinsed with boiling water.

Ask how various dishes are prepared. Well-educated restaurants provide their servers with specific information, and they will, if necessary, ask the chef for more details. The server is, remember, your link to the kitchen.

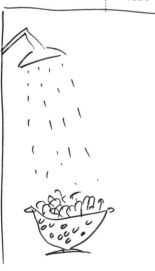

Ask for your salad with the dressing on the side, too. Many a server will nod vigorously when you do because it's such a common request. And while you're at it, select a dressing that is not one of those thick, creamy ones. An oil and vinegar dressing is better, and best of all is simply to ask for the oil and vinegar so that you can make your own dressing and use less oil.

Ask that butter be left off (even a grilled entrée may arrive swimming in butter that has been put on top after it's cooked) and that sauces be served on the side. Rather than immediately dumping the sauce onto your food, try using just a little bit for flavor, maybe dipping the fork in it so that you get a taste with the food. This is called taking charge of your life.

Ask, too, how the vegetables are prepared. If preparation involves the use of olive oil, you can ask them to go easy. If preparation involves butter or rich sauces, you can ask to have the vegetables steamed. Maybe the server will tell you sorry, it's too late, they're made in advance, in which case simply ask if they could be put into a colander and rinsed with boiling water.

Once your order has been placed, your conversation with the server may not be over. In spite of your best efforts, when your food arrives, it might not be exactly what you asked for.

◆   ◆   ◆   ◆

In the old days, when you went to a restaurant with a group of people and your order came out well done when you'd asked for it rare, well, maybe you said something and maybe you didn't. It might have been the case that only the members of your party who had the word "obnoxious" tattooed on their foreheads would think of sending back their food, a gesture that was perceived as unpleasant, disruptive, and, in general, antisocial.

Now you have more at stake. If there is something the matter with your order, you'll want to say so. There are, of course, ways to do this. A not so fine line exists between "assertive" and "aggressive"; assertive is the way to go. Think of this as taking care of yourself, rather than an attempt to win the Most Offensive award.

You don't have to make a big deal of the fact that even though you asked for no butter, you could spot your order shimmering at twenty paces. You simply say quietly to the server, "I'm sorry to have to ask you to take this back, but I did order it without butter." There's no need to be embarrassed. If those in your group elect to make a major production out of this, then they, not you, deserve to be embarrassed.

Salad Bars

A few words about salad bars. They get a lot of mileage out of their name. If they were called, say, "glop stops," they wouldn't attract much business. But, in fact, glop stops is a great deal more descriptive of what they really are.

"I'm sorry to have to ask you to take this back, but I did order it without butter."

*As a rule,
the heavier
the salad
bar item, the
higher the
fat content.*

The average salad bar has a large bowl of lettuce, lying on top of which is a pair of tongs, cleverly designed so that when you pick up a generous portion of lettuce leaves, most of them fall back into the bowl before you can get them on your plate. And then there are all those people behind you in line, and, well, you just have to keep moving.

What you move on to are a series of cold concoctions that are, more often than not, loaded with fat and calories. You'll find potato salad, cole slaw, macaroni salad in a creamy dressing. You'll find chopped egg (it's the yolks that contain fat, but if you try to pick out the whites here, you'll cause a riot), grated cheese (contains fat), mushrooms soaking in oil, and more. You'll also find tomatoes, fresh mushrooms, cucumbers, onions, peppers, pickled beets, and other typical salad ingredients. Here you are, holding up the line, and you have to think fast. In fact, it's quite simple. As a rule, the heavier the salad bar item, the higher the fat content (with the exception of carrots and beets). Think what you'd put in ye olde salade bowle if you were fixing an ordinary salad at home, go forth, and do likewise.

At the end of the bar you'll see vats of various salad dressings, sometimes identified, sometimes not, and even when they are identified you might not realize it because the signs are sitting on top of the plastic cover of the salad bar, not exactly in your line of sight. The thicker dressings come in creamy white, tan, even pink. There is probably a brown, oil-based dressing there, too. Whatever their color, THESE DRESSINGS ARE FULL OF FAT, unless they are labeled otherwise. Incidentally, those long-handled ladles that hang over the edge of the dressing containers hold two tablespoons of dressing, which, if labeled, would announce the sad fact that *they contain close to 20 grams of fat.*

The dressings can be a fine addition to a salad, greatly improving the chances that you'll eat and enjoy it. So use some, not a lot, maybe about one fourth of a ladleful.

Better to use the oil and vinegar that you'll find in the two little bottles sure to be around there someplace. Or (okay, this is asking a lot) just splash some vinegar on top and feel incredibly virtuous.

Bread and Butter

While you're waiting for your food to come, you'll notice that bread (or rolls) and butter have been brought to the table. Many times they take the form of buttery rolls and garlic bread. It is sort of a knee-jerk reaction to consume large portions while you have a nice conversation and perhaps a glass of wine.

Ask the server for plain bread, and eat it without the butter that will be served attractively in little pots, or in little candy shapes, or in a ball that looks like a scoop of ice cream. If you are in the habit of using butter, you'll probably want to put it out of arm's reach, admittedly not easy when you consider the size of some of the tables in restaurants these days. The idea is to be fully aware of what you're eating, rather than awaken from a trance to find that you aren't very hungry, what with the entire loaf of garlic bread in your stomach.

Serving Size

You really have no control over restaurant serving sizes. You take what you get, and it's usually more than you need. Pasta may be served in a hubcap. If it tastes good, you eat all of it. Even if it doesn't taste wonderful, the old tapes play in your head – "Clean your plate! People are starving all over the world!" – and you finish anyway, loosening your belt as you do so. (It's that "rounder and rounder" thing again.)

There are options. You can divide the portion and ask to have part of it wrapped to take home. You can offer some to others in your group. If neither of these works (maybe you're on your way to a party and don't want to leave food sitting in the car half the night; maybe there are no tak-

> ### THE LAST RESORT:
>
> Pick up the salt shaker and, with a last look around, put on so much salt that the food becomes inedible. That way, you won't sit there and pick, pick, pick until you suddenly notice that you've eaten the whole thing, even though you had no intention of doing so. A no-fail way to limit serving size.

ers for your leftovers), you have a last resort. We've tried it and guarantee that it works. (See box on previous page.)

Dessert

You don't need to read here that fresh fruit is the best possible dessert pick because you already know that. If you absolutely must have a sweet dessert, make it something like fruit pie, but not à la mode. Remember that "la mode" – the fashion – these days is to cut down on things like ice cream. See if you can get someone to split a piece of pie with you. That way, unless you are on the attack, you will eat only half. You'll eat even less if your companion is on the attack. If you can manage to avoid eating the crust, the fattiest part of the pie, so much the better. Otherwise, try eating just half of it.

The ever-popular dessert tray makes life all the more difficult because you can see what you're missing, and that's no accident. Apparently the word is out that restaurant patrons who see "mocha whipped cream torte" printed on a menu may pass it up, but they may not be able to resist upon seeing the dessert itself. The server arrives with the dessert tray and describes each delectable offering in such detail that you can feel yourself gaining weight just by listening. But do your best to stay away from rich pastries and other creamy things, which are nothing more than morsels (granted, tasty morsels) of fat and calories – and what most people imagine when the word "dessert" comes into the conversation. Instead, try one of the fruit ices that are popular, so popular, in fact, they are being called "sorbets," which just goes

> **THINK "MIX AND MATCH" AGAIN**
>
> If there is a raspberry purée over the chocolate cheesecake, and they also offer fresh strawberries, ask if you might have strawberries with the raspberry purée. Or, if they have no fruit listed, ask. It may be available as an appetizer and they will serve it to you for dessert.

to show how classy things sound in French. Frequently they are homemade and are a refreshing end to the meal.

An old diet expression says, "A minute on the lips, a lifetime on the hips." That thinking works here, too. If you give in and eat that rich, creamy, chocolate dessert, it's gone in a minute, but the effects linger in your body. The rhyme may be lost, but the idea isn't. And it's not just your hips, it's your heart.

Coffee and Tea

If you like a good cup of coffee or fragrant tea and must lighten it, ask for milk instead of cream. Make it low-fat milk if they have it, which they probably won't, but if enough people ask for it, you can be sure they'll get it eventually. Don't be fooled into thinking that nondairy creamers are better; their big advantage is to shopkeepers since they don't spoil, but they may contain a lot of fat.

A glass of sparkling water with a lemon or lime wedge also makes a nice ending for the meal. If it is served in one of those great-looking glasses that restaurants are investing in, it will seem to taste all the better.

Lunch

When you are really and truly watching your food intake, one of the day-to-day problems you will face is lunch. Of course you've always thought of lunch as a meal, not a problem, but it can be both a meal and a problem.

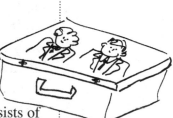

The difficulty comes when you work in an office and lunch consists of a fast bite somewhere. Since fast bites are generally high in fat, the solution is to carry your lunch with you.

Now it may well be that the last time you carried your lunch it was in a lunch box with your favorite cartoon character painted all over it, and a small thermos bottle tucked inside it whose glass liner broke and had to be replaced every week. (Could it have been because you played catch with it on the school bus?)

If you're feeling a little crazy, you might buy yourself a new lunch box. Lunch boxes are still around, but the thermos bottles have an unbreakable plastic lining. Your old favorite cartoon friends may be gone, but you'll find an enormous selection of possible replacements.

Strategies

for

Eating Out

Undoubtedly it has already occurred to you that you do not need a lunch box in order to carry your lunch. You can use anything from a brown bag (simple but nice) to an attaché case (upscale and trendy). The issue is what to take in it.

To a great extent, this will depend on where you are going to be doing your eating. If you'll be staying at your desk, is there a microwave oven nearby? This would allow you to pack leftovers from last night's dinner; they could be reheated quickly and easily. If you have no access to a microwave, or if you are of the persuasion that you'll glow in the dark if you get too close to one, think "cold food." Maybe those same leftovers.

Lunch: Sandwiches

The most obvious cold lunch is a sandwich, and what makes a sandwich a sandwich is, of course, bread. Depending on which of the amazing variety of breads you choose, sandwiches can take on many different personalities – spicy, seeded, soft, crusty. Some even have vegetables baked in them. The bakery section of the supermarket is loaded with these wonderful breads, many of which are made with no fat.

You can always use bagels. "A sandwich from a bagel?" you are thinking. If that sounds just a little too Whopper-sized for you, consider eating a salad with a bagel on the side. You can keep bagels on hand in the freezer. (Hint: Slice them before freezing. Slicing a frozen bagel is so difficult and dangerous that it could be an Olympic event. A sliced frozen bagel is easier to toast, too.)

The flat, round pocket bread known as pita is another option. Widely available, this no-fat-added bread comes in white and whole wheat, and in two sizes, the larger of which is easier to use for sandwiches. If you cut the bread in half, you have two half-circles with an opening, a pocket, exposed.

Whatever bread you have chosen, you now have the task of turning it into a sandwich. Cartoon character Dagwood Bumstead, an expert sandwich-maker, popularized the enormous, jaw-dislocating version a long time ago, and the concept lives on. It's worth bearing in mind, however, that the ideal sandwich isn't too big to bite into.

Besides, Dagwood was lucky. He looked the same year in and year out, no matter how big his sandwiches were. Real people, however, get rounder and rounder.

If, when you think of sandwiches, you immediately start envisioning deli meats, at least envision fat-free deli meats. Then, instead of piling up the meat, try using less and making up the difference with those vegetables that come in nice jars, and are waiting for you at the grocery store. Red peppers, for example, are made without oil.

Or you might make a tuna salad using one of those little cans of water-packed, rather than oil-packed, tuna. The two varieties sit side by side on your grocer's shelf, and you just have to

> ### FOR A REAL TREAT
>
> Instead of tuna, try a bit of cold salmon from last night's Salmon Cooked in Foil (see recipe, page 203) or maybe some leftover Grilled Turkey Breast (see recipe, page 199).

make sure you pick up the right one. If you've still got some oil-packed tuna in your cupboard, or if you find that you grabbed the wrong one after all, dump it into a strainer and run cold water over it. You'll get rid of most of the oil.

Drain the tuna as you would do normally, and mix it with chopped onion or peppers, maybe some shredded carrot and a bit of horseradish for spice, whatever you like. (Better skip the onions if you've got a big post-lunch meeting scheduled.) Instead of using mayonnaise, or even low-fat or fat-free mayonnaise, try a bit of mustard (one that contains no oil) mixed with fat-free yogurt (see recipe for Yogurt-Mustard Sauce, page 191. Or see recipe for Crunchy Tuna Salad, page 181).

Now add some romaine lettuce – it fits more easily if you first cut it up or pull it apart – add the tuna, and you're all set.

You can make a salad sandwich by cutting up any vegetables you like – carrots, celery, radishes, cucumbers, peppers, onions, tomatoes, and so on. (Is it true that tomatoes are really fruits? Inquiring minds want to know.) You could put in marinated beans and vegetables (see recipe for Marinated Beans and Vegetables, page 185). Sprouts are delicious with this. Should you be under the impression that sprouts are for antiestab-

Strategies

for

Eating Out

Pancakes or waffles (without butter) are a better choice than muffins, croissants, and doughnuts.

lishment-vegetarian-hippie types, guess again. They are very tasty and add a nice texture to the contents of the sandwich. (You can grow sprouts or buy them at the supermarket. Once upon a time, we did the former. Now we do the latter.) Stuff the mixture into the pita, and drizzle over it that Yogurt-Mustard Sauce mentioned a minute ago.

Eating Out for Breakfast

Y ou may have noticed that eating out for breakfast hasn't been discussed. The brutal fact is that breakfast foods tend to be high, often very high, in fat: eggs, bacon, sausage, et cetera, et cetera, et cetera. If you find yourself eating breakfast in a restaurant, you can always order oatmeal, but not everyone considers it a big treat. If you want More Traditional Breakfast Fare, you can cut your losses by ordering pancakes or waffles without that dollop of butter on top, and then use syrup. (You might even add some cut-up fresh fruit.) In fact, pancakes or waffles are a better choice than muffins, croissants, and doughnuts, which are generally loaded with fat.

Another possibility is to order an egg substitute or an egg white omelet. This can then be filled with peppers, mushrooms, tomatoes, onions, whatever, but not cheese. It's worth keeping in mind that restaurants offering egg white omelets have to do something with the yolks, and chances are extremely good that what they do with them is add them to the regular omelet mixture, thereby increasing the fat content of those omelets.

Restaurants frequently use plastic squeeze bottles of margarine and squirt it in pans and on the grill when they prepare food. Obviously this adds a lot of fat to whatever food is cooked there. So you'll want to ask that your omelet be prepared without fat on the grill. This won't affect preparation, because the grill is already seasoned and the omelet won't stick.

Order a bagel, an English muffin, or toast, dry (no butter or margarine), and spread it with jam or honey.

Business Lunches and Dinners

There are times when your work involves a meal with a lot of other people, and the food has been ordered ahead of time. Maybe you had a little input ("Please check one: Chicken with Cream Sauce, Fried Fish Fillet"), but you understandably feel as though the food is pretty much out of your control at this point.

Not true! When you find that you'll be going to a restaurant or hotel for a meeting, don't be afraid to call ahead, speak to the catering department, and simply explain the situation. Most likely you'll be pleasantly surprised to find that the kitchen will be very accommodating, and will modify the menu to suit your needs.

Fast Food

A fast word on fast food restaurants. They boast an enormous wall menu that offers very little in the way of low-fat foods. Fish, normally considered low in fat, is not among them, being almost invariably breaded and fried. Here are your choices:

- Grilled, not breaded, chicken sandwich (plain, not deluxe)
- Grilled chicken salad
- Junior hamburger (3 ounces, and hold the creamy sauces, cheese, etc.)

Speaking of salad, the dressing comes in a little packet made of a material that is almost impossible to tear open. Which turns out to be just as well, because, unless the dressing is low fat or fat free, you're better off using none at all. One packet contains up to 21 grams of fat, and chances are you use more than one.

What else can you find to eat? Potatoes, but not fries. A baked potato is fine (if they have it), but order it plain; the fat hangs out in the toppings. Probably the closest thing you'll find to a vegetable is a side salad, not an interesting one at that, and you've just read the bad news about the dressing.

Pizza is another type of fast food that is high in fat, thanks to the meat, the cheese, and the oil. However, many places will make you a meatless, no-cheese pizza, easy on the oil. If you ask. They might even add vegetables. If you ask again. And who knows? Maybe they'll name the pizza after you!

Strategies

for

Eating Out

Don't be afraid to call ahead and speak to the catering department.

Strategies

for

Eating Out

If, say, you are traveling by airplane, take a couple of fat-free bagels, as well as apples or bananas, along for the ride.

It's worth taking the time to find fast food places that offer low-fat choices. Once you've found them, they'll be yours forever.

For the Healthy Traveler

In today's busy world, it is essential that you not get so hungry you grab anything handy, loaded with fat though it may be. When you are hungry, your goal is simply to fill your stomach, and only later do you reconsider, and regret, what you had to eat. It's a shame to fill yourself with fat-laden food that, most likely, doesn't taste very good anyway.

When you are traveling, you need something to tide you over until you can get some real food. If, say, you are traveling by airplane, take a couple of bagels, as well as apples or bananas, along for the ride. Bagels have the advantage of being extremely portable, and they aren't messy, either. Chances are that it will be a long time until food service, and you'll have a good, filling, not particularly messy snack to munch on. Then, when the airline "food" (the term is used loosely) finally arrives, you won't be forced to eat it just because you are so hungry you're ready to eat the seat in front of you. Instead you can pick and choose from your food tray. There will probably be a salad (try to go easy on the dressing), and a roll, which you can eat without butter (or whatever "spread" they offer, congratulating themselves for avoiding butter).

If the airline food falls into the "inedible" category, you can whip out a package of fat-free dehydrated soup (tasty soups are made by Nile Spice, Fantastic Foods[26], and Knorr, for example). It comes packaged in such a way that you add hot water (ask for some when the beverage service comes around) and eat it directly from the container the soup comes in. Handy. Disposable. Give it a try.

If you give them at least twenty-four hours' notice, airlines will provide a "special meal" for you. Your best bet is to request a diabetic meal (yes! really!) or a fresh fruit plate, tastier than the "low-fat" meals offered. We should mention that we have had a fair amount of experience with special meals that somehow never materialized, so don't assume you'll get one even if you requested it. ("When exactly did you order the meal?" we've been asked by the flight attendant. Were we paranoid in thinking she imagined herself in the company of a pathological liar?)

Maybe you are traveling to another country, where you'll be eating in restaurants. You might not be able to read the menu, and if you can't read it, you probably can't talk to the server, either. Here are some tips so you can at least steer clear of saturated fat:

HOW TO SAY, "PLEASE – NO CREAM, NO CHEESE, NO BUTTER," IN FOUR LANGUAGES.

FRENCH: S'il vous plaît ["seel voo play"]–sans ["sahn"] crème ["crem"], sans ["sahn"] fromage ["fro-mahj"], sans ["sahn"] beurre ["burr"].

SPANISH: Por favor ["poor fa-vour"]–sin ["sing"] crema ["crema"], sin ["sing"] queso ["kay-so"], sin ["sing"] mantequilla ["mant-a-key-a"].

GERMAN: Bitte ["bit-uh"]–keine ["kine-uh"] Sahne ["sa-nuh"], kein ["kine"] Käse ["kayz-uh"], keine ["kine-uh"] Butter ["boot-er"].

ITALIAN: Per ["pair"] favore ["fa-vor-ay"]–niente ["nee-en-tay"] crema ["cray-ma"], niente ["nee-en-tay"] formaggio ["for-mah-jo"], niente ["nee-en-tay"] burro ["boor-o"].

Eating at Someone's House

At a restaurant you can order whatever you want, which wouldn't go over very well at a dinner party, where the custom is to eat the food you're served, fat and all.

However, friends will take notice if you have developed a distinctive eating style. The fact that it is your chief subject of conversation may have something to do with it. If you were a vegetarian, a friend inviting you to a small dinner party would probably have you in mind when the menu was planned, and the same holds true here.

Yes, if this is just a few good friends getting together, you'll do fine. For one thing, your host may run the menu by you when the invitation is extended. For another, you can make simple requests at that time: Might some dressing be kept aside for your salad, so that you can add it your-

Strategies

for

Eating Out

*Have
something to
eat before
going to big
parties.*

self? And might some bread be left unbuttered for you? Then, too, you can offer to bring dessert, and bring a low-fat one.

Big Parties

The problem is with big parties, huge parties, weddings, and the key is to eat first. That's right, you're on your way out to dinner but you eat before you go. There's no need to sit down to a full-course meal, or to use a cloth napkin, but the idea is that you shouldn't be hungry when you get to this food fest. It's much easier to turn down the fried cheese balls being passed when you aren't in the first stages of starvation.

Life is a little easier if this is a buffet. You can take what you want and be spared that "pushing around" thing we all learned to do when we were kids and our plates were contaminated by peas.

Anyway, if the fare is spread out before you at a buffet table, count yourself lucky. And if someone is serving, so much the better, because you can ask casually what in the world this stuff is.

But there are those elegant dinner parties where the food is passed to you at the table, and you help yourself, putting it on a dinner plate the size of a sombrero. Here comes the crab in cream sauce, the beef already coated with bearnaise sauce, the broccoli lost in hollandaise sauce. Here are the potatoes with butter and cheese, the already-buttered rolls. It's lonely at the top.

But forge ahead as best you can, keeping in mind that you have to live in this world. You can take small portions, claiming that you spoiled your appetite by eating too many of those delicious – what were they? Oh, yes, of course! – fried cheese balls. Help yourself to a little bit of a couple of things, and surreptitiously scrape off as much of the sauce as you can manage without appearing to be playing with your food. Forget the rolls.

Dessert will undoubtedly be some rich something, and if you can bear to turn it down, do. If not, try to eat just a bit of it, and focus on what is sure to be the best cup of coffee since the Folger's people first pawned off instant coffee on unsuspecting restaurant patrons.

Develop a secret smile that you can use when other guests marvel at how little you eat. You, of course, are stuffed to the gills, having eaten at home, and you've had some extra goodies at this party.

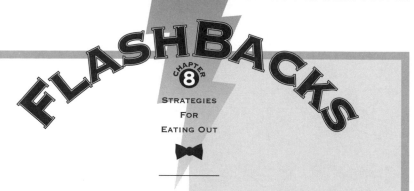

FLASHBACKS

CHAPTER 8

STRATEGIES
FOR
EATING OUT

☞ Take lunch to work.

☞ **If you eat at restaurants frequently,** you can't consider every restaurant meal a special event.

☞ **Talk to the server:**
- Ask how various dishes are prepared.
- Ask for "no cream, no cheese, no butter."
- Order foods broiled or grilled rather than fried.
- Ask that salad dressings be served on the side.

☞ **Study the menu:**
- Avoid dishes that have "cream" in the name or description, or that say "pan-fried," "crispy," "au gratin," or "scalloped."
- "Mix and match" to make the perfect meal.
- Choose fresh fruit, sorbet, or fruit pie (go easy on the crust) instead of rich, creamy deserts.

☞ **Stay away from fat- and oil-laden dishes at the salad bar.**

☞ Eat something at home before going out to a dinner party. **Don't go hungry!**

Chapter Nine Strategies for Eating In

Strategies

for

Eating In

"When Mama Got 'The Consciousness'"
– Deborah Levy

The year was 1988. Well, actually it was 1987, but it wasn't until '88 that we realized what had happened. Daddy was on a special low-fat diet for his heart, and Mama had sacrificed good cooking of her own free will. She devoted her kitchen time to making cardboard taste good. Though it was Daddy who was on the diet, it was Mama who became a fanatic. When she got The Consciousness, no one was safe. Not only family members, but friends, acquaintances, and people at neighboring tables in restaurants got the benefit of her wisdom. Up and down the East Coast, Mama preached the evils of red meat, heavy cream, and egg yolks.

None of us realized just how far she had gone until June, when we gave a cocktail party. As my brother and I were making a list of things to get (cheese and crackers, nuts) Mama looked at us as if we'd gone insane. "Nobody eats that stuff anymore," she informed us. It was evident that she felt we had failed her. But she valiantly took our education in hand and explained the need for celery, carrots, and a dip made from fat-free yogurt. My brother and I looked at each other in despair.

How To Cope With Family Rebellion

Just try to do something that's good for your family, and they'll turn against you every time, particularly when it involves a change of eating habits. Too bad, because while it's well and good to go out to dinner once in awhile (Well and good? It's the best), more often than not you'll find yourself eating at home with the family.

Eating in. The opposite of eating out, in more ways than one, especially if you're in charge of meal planning, shopping, preparation, and cleanup.

Strategies

for

Eating In

Eating in may well involve other family members, small family members, kids. As it happens, one of the things that makes kids what they are is their resistance to change, at least when it has to do with the way things have always been done at home. Many's the child who greeted Mother's new hairdo with "Yuk! I liked the old way better!" and other equally endearing remarks. Or reacted with dismay upon discovering a new brand of dishwashing liquid on the counter, not that the child ever washes the dishes, mind you.

It comes as no surprise to hear that a great many youngsters are not what you'd call interested in trying new things to eat. You may have to introduce a child to a new food as many as *fourteen times* before it is familiar enough to really eat, not just pick at.[27] Children vastly prefer foods that are instantly recognizable, not to mention overwhelmingly familiar, in both appearance and taste. Their idea of gourmet runs to the sorts of things that sponsor Saturday morning cartoon shows.

Now that a new day is dawning for you in the area of food preparation, you're undoubtedly aware that Junior may not take kindly to the requisite changes. Perhaps you can already envision the dinner table conversation:

"Ugh! What's this?"

"How can you say 'Ugh' when you haven't even taken a bite yet?"

"And I'm not taking a bite, either. No way! I want fried chicken!"

Be grateful if that's Junior talking, not your spouse.

So how *can* you cope with family rebellion? First of all by dealing with your own. And you may very well be feeling rebellious, what with having to change the way you've been doing things in the kitchen lo these many years. You must be convinced of the worth of this. After all, what could be more important than protecting your family and yourself? Recognizing this will serve as fortification against complaints such as the one mentioned a minute ago. Get the family involved! Have them pick their favorite recipes from the back of this book, and you can all fix them together.

When you know you want to protect your family, your family will come to know it, too, and will appreciate your efforts in the end. In the meantime, give yourself credit for trying.

CHAPTER
9

Strategies

for

Eating In

How To Make Changes That Will Win Your Family's Heart

R emember that you are not alone in this effort, because there are an enormous number of products on the market that can help you in your shift to low-fat cooking, more products all the time. But even with this kind of help, you may harbor fears about slaving over a hot stove only to have noses turn up at the dishes you've prepared. You may picture yourself lecturing about children who go to bed hungry every night, even as you are dimly aware that this tactic is hardly designed to win anybody over. But what *is* the best way to win them over? For one thing, don't make a big deal about all of this. There's no need to give a major address on the subject of eating healthfully, ending with something like, "You can bet your boots there are going to be some changes around here, folks!" Such an approach is guaranteed to draw the battle lines, which you'd clearly rather not do. Milk is a good place to begin quietly reducing fat in the family diet. If the family is used to drinking whole milk (in which half the calories come from fat), switch first to "reduced fat" (formerly 2%), which still packs a lot of fat, then to "low fat" (formerly 1%), and finally to "fat-free" (formerly skim). We know, we know. Compared to whole milk, this tastes watery. But once the family is used to low-fat milk, it won't taste much different. *(Note: Discuss any changes in diet with your pediatrician. Young children should not reduce fat the way older people should.)*

Milk is a good place to begin quietly reducing fat in the family diet.

You can introduce new foods gradually, too. Don't suddenly present things so wildly different from the usual fare that those gathered around the dinner table will wonder if this is their house. You might want to make some of the "embarrassingly simple" recipes in this book (beginning on page 137), and start by serving them along with other dishes that your family eats all the time. As you move away from the familiar, bring in reinforcements, serving plenty of pasta or rice or potatoes, plenty of fresh vegetables, and a good loaf of bread.

Chicken, the Transition Food

We are a chicken-eating country. That's good, because, unless the chicken is fried (sorry, Junior), it's a low-fat choice. Even people who are not trying to eat a healthier diet are accidentally doing just that when they eat baked or broiled chicken.

Even though it's better to eat chicken than a different part of the cow every night, eating a lot of chicken is not a goal, not an end in itself. It is not The Ideal Entrée because there is no such thing, variety being the key.

But because chicken has broad-based appeal, can be prepared in so many ways, and is low in fat, it may be seen as a kind of "transition food," with the ability to move Americans in the direction of healthier eating. "Embarrassingly simple" chicken recipes begin on page 192.

By the way, have you noticed that Kentucky Fried Chicken is taking advantage of chicken's link with good health, and now calls itself KFC? Are we supposed to forget what that stands for? If the Colonel had made his fortune touting Kentucky Broiled Chicken, you can bet your drumstick they wouldn't be using initials today.

Now here's an interesting little tidbit about turkey, chicken's cousin when it comes to "transition food." An article in the Tunica Times, in Tunica, Mississippi,[28] tells how to deep fry a turkey. That's right, deep fry. This is not, repeat NOT, a misprint. Rosemary Tindle, a Home Economist, suggests using a small turkey (12-15 pounds) and putting it in a pot big enough to completely

> ### DON'T FORGET ABOUT TURKEY
>
> A couple of hints:
>
> - There's no need to wait until Thanksgiving to serve turkey. Every once in a while, cook a fresh turkey breast, lower in fat than the rest of the turkey, and much easier to prepare (either roast it or see recipe for Grilled Turkey Breast, page 199).
>
> - If you decide to use ground turkey as a replacement for hamburger, be sure to buy ground turkey *breast*. If you don't, you'll be eating meat that has skin ground up in it, and the result will be not only fatty but pretty gruesome to contemplate.

Strategies

for

Eating In

Snow
Chicken

▼

submerge the turkey in oil. How much oil? About 2 1/2 to 3 gallons, she says. This strikes us as pretty hazardous, well beyond the article's acknowledged danger of "hot, popping oil."

It's not the food itself that makes a difference. It's the preparation.

Chicken: Recipe Ideas

Rather than turn you loose and back to KFC, we offer (in addition to the "embarrassingly simple" chicken recipes beginning on page 192) several fast, easy, low-fat chicken recipe ideas. Note that these are only ideas, around which you can build your own recipes if you wish. Use skinless chicken.

■ Marinate breasts in fat-free bottled dressing, to which you've added chopped onion and garlic. Cook on the grill, which, by the way, can be used all year round. Never use it indoors, though, because it gives off noxious fumes. If there's snow on the ground, no problem. If there's snow on the grill, brush it off. Grilled food is delicious – "Snow Chicken" – and you can get away with using a lot less fat. (Don't blacken the food, though, because charred food is not particularly good for you to eat.)

■ Cut chicken into strips before marinating and cooking on the grill. (Or use chicken "tenders," small pieces of chicken breast that you'll find in the supermarket with the other poultry.) Add to pasta. You might also sauté zucchini in a tiny bit of olive oil (one teaspoon per serving, tops) and add that, too. Finish with a good tomato sauce.

■ Cut up uncooked chicken and stir-fry with vegetables in a bit of oil (one teaspoon per serving, tops). A little chicken goes a long way.

■ Poach chicken in a small amount of chicken broth. Add onion, carrot, and celery (without the chicken skin, you'll need some help to create flavor). By the way, if you are using canned broth that is not fat free, store it in the refrigerator. Why clutter up your already-crowded refrigerator with canned broth? Because fat congeals on the top of the refrigerated broth, and you can just scrape off the fat and have fat-free broth.

■ After the above chicken is poached, remove vegetables and purée them in a food processor to serve with the chicken. Season to taste, and serve over rice or couscous (little pasta bits that kids love).

A Typical Non-Chicken Meal
Meatballs

Low-fat meals need not feature chicken, of course. Or turkey, for that matter. Even in the most extreme fat-consuming households, the change can be easy and subtle. The trick is to start with the most acceptable dish (from the standpoint of this new way of eating) that has been served routinely, and go from there.

Say that the most acceptable dish is spaghetti and meatballs made with an old family recipe for tomato sauce. (Let's hope you're not dousing it with old-fashioned grated cheese.) First, the meatballs. Are you using the very leanest ground beef you can buy? (Keep in mind that the amount of fat in ground beef labeled "Lean" varies from store to store, and you probably won't even find an "Extra Lean" label. So look for 10 grams of fat, 4.5 grams of saturated fat OR LESS! If there's no label, you'll have to check with the butcher. Or buy ground sirloin.) You can further reduce fat by replacing some of the ground meat with bread crumbs.

When you cook the meatballs, do you sort of fry them in their own fat? If you do, instead try putting them under the broiler so that the fat will run off. (Remember to turn them so they will brown on all sides.)

Sauce

Now the sauce. What's in that "old family recipe"? (In case your old family didn't make pasta sauce, or if you'd rather not bother, there are a number of fat-free choices on the market. Some are in jars. Contadina Tomato Basil Sauce is very good and is refrigerated.)

If you do make your own sauce and the only fat is a little olive oil, you're all right. (Remember, one teaspoon per serving.) But if the recipe includes pork fat and other unacceptable ingredients, work on adapting the recipe. Anyone who makes tomato sauce from scratch is not a rank amateur as far as cooking is concerned, so you're sure to be clever enough and

Strategies

for

Eating In

*If there is a
puddle of
dressing
sitting in the
bottom, then
you like
your salad
well soaked.
Consider
using one of
the many
fat-free
versions
now
available.*

inventive enough to re-work the fat content of the dish. You may want to add more mushrooms, onions, garlic, or herbs to replace the flavor that is lost when you take out the fat.

Bread

Do you serve garlic bread with this meal? If you buy it frozen, check the label. You'll be amazed at how much fat it has. If you make it yourself, don't bother. You're better off serving a nice hot, crusty loaf of bread, and it's especially good for sopping up that tomato sauce everybody's so crazy about.

Salad

It's likely that a salad accompanies this particular meal. A word about their dressings.

Salads live and die by their dressings. When delicately coated, the greens are supreme; when covered, they are overpowered. You'll know which way you fix your salads by what's left in the bowl when the salad is gone. If there is a puddle of dressing sitting in the bottom, then you like your salad well soaked. Consider using one of the many fat-free versions now available, although odds are you won't be absolutely crazy about the taste or the smell or the appearance. These dressings do, however, serve the purpose. And they make terrific marinades.

If the empty salad bowl is almost dry or is glistening, you obviously don't use a lot of dressing, preferring to taste the salad as well as the dressing. You might be surprised when we suggest that the best way to do that is to use a regular dressing – not reduced fat, not fat free. It tastes wonderful, smells wonderful, looks wonderful – and contains more fat per serving than we've been recommending. We feel that's a small price to pay if it means you are eating vegetable-filled salads.

You have two embarrassingly

> **OUR FAVORITE HOMEMADE:**
>
> Put 1/4 cup olive oil, 1/8 cup red wine or balsamic vinegar, and 1 teaspoon Dijon mustard in a small jar. Shake well. That's it. Enough for a salad for four.

simple options when it comes to delicious dressings: homemade (see box on previous page) and ready-made.

Ready-made: Shake bottle, unscrew cap, and pour.

Dessert

When it comes to dessert, change is more difficult, and you'll meet with opposition if your family's idea of dessert has meant a sweet treat at the end of every meal.

One change involves making the sweet an occasional treat. Another involves checking the Dessert section of this book (beginning on page 209) and finding a low-fat sweet.

Yet another change involves choosing other sorts of desserts. Try to stick to fruit – fresh, dried, even canned (in its own juice rather than in heavy syrup). (See fruit recipes, beginning on page 210.) Summertime offers wonderful fresh fruits such as melons and berries, which combine to make a delicious fruit bowl. In winter, oranges and grapefruit can be sectioned. For company, put the sections with their juice in a bowl, add some cut-up strawberries, and mix in a bit of orange-flavored liqueur. You can put A Great Raspberry Sauce over the fruit, too (see recipe, page 220).

If you want to serve something baked, best of all is angel food cake, which contains no fat. You can serve it with fruit, or you can slice the cake in half, crosswise, and spread fruit topping between the layers. Or add unsweetened cocoa powder during baking, resulting in chocolate flavor without the fat found in chocolate (see recipe for "Chocolate" Birthday Cake, page 227).

Presentation

As you think about new ways of preparing food, think, too, about the way it looks on the plate.

Imagine on your white dinner plate: a piece of poached flounder flanked by a baked potato and a helping of mashed turnips, with perhaps a crusty piece of bread on the side. Sounds like a healthy, low-fat meal, which is what we've been discussing this whole time, haven't we, for heaven's sake? Ah, but think about how the dinner looks. It may remind

Strategies

for

Eating In

*Think of
steamed
vegetables
as a "bed"
for your
chicken or
fish.*

you of the picture you "drew" when you were a kid, a blank sheet of paper that you said was a polar bear in a snowstorm. Well, in fact the flounder/potato/turnip/bread might be just as hard to locate on that white dinner plate. It may taste good, but you start off with a couple of strikes against you in the presentation department.

In other words, you aren't taking advantage of the possibilities of advertising the meal you've just prepared. Short of investing in colored plates, admittedly a possible, if extravagant, solution, you'll want to begin to consider: ❶color; ❷texture; ❸garnish; and ❹arrangement of food.

An attractive plate of food contains a variety of colors. There is almost always something in the pink/red/orange/yellow group (salmon? red beets? red beans? tomatoes? sweet potatoes? carrots?); something in the green group (spinach? broccoli? asparagus? green beans? lima beans? artichoke? peas?); and something in the white or brown group (pasta? rice? potato? meat? chicken? fish?).

Variety in texture is also pleasant, which is why you probably wouldn't serve mashed potatoes and mashed carrots at the same meal, unless you were trying out some new piece of kitchen equipment and got carried away.

Contrary to popular opinion, restaurants don't have the exclusive right to garnish a dinner plate. Maybe you don't want to bother

> **HOT TIP:**
>
> You won't stick to this new way of eating for the rest of your life if the food doesn't look appealing and appetizing.

with rosettes and things, but try steaming some carrot "coins" or slivered carrots just to put on the plate to add some color. You can do the same with purple cabbage. If you're in a hurry (and who isn't?), don't even bother cooking them first. They'll still add the color and serve the purpose. You can eat them uncooked, too.

Finally, the way you arrange food on the plate can enhance both the appearance of the food and the pleasure of eating it, so take a few seconds to make things look attractive. Consider a "stacking" effect, putting the grilled salmon on top of the spinach rather than next to it, the way they do in those fancy restaurants. Or julienne some zucchini and yellow squash in the food processor, steam gently, and put that underneath the

Strategies

for

Eating In

fish or chicken or whatever. In other words, think of the vegetable as a "bed." Or put the salmon on top of a pool of Yogurt-Mustard Sauce (see recipe, page 191). You'll make the plate look beautiful, with no added effort. An unbeatable combination.

There is definitely more to eating than putting food in your mouth. Interestingly, the Japanese consider all of this so important that their country's dietary guidelines state that experiences related to eating must be pleasurable. And if you fill all the senses, you'll be less likely to overeat.

Moving On

It's a lot easier to talk about eating low fat than it is to maintain a low-fat way of eating. Sometimes it seems as if everything is against you. In fact, when we were writing an early draft of this book on the computer, merrily cutting and pasting away, the computer merged two sections accidentally, and the following sentences came out of the printer. This is true, really. We swear it. Besides, who could make up something like this?

> If you are feeling creative, ask the butcher to take the bone out and the skin off of a turkey breast. When you get home and take it out of the package, it won't look wildly appetizing, but don't despair. Rinse it in cold water, pat dry with paper towels, then cut some slashes in it and put it in a roasting pan. *Stick some cloves of garlic in the slashes, dump a little lemon juice in there, too, and rub the whole thing with pork fat and other unacceptable ingredients* [italics added].

So here you are, providing nutritious and, you hope, delicious meals for your family, meeting with occasional resistance nevertheless ("How come we never have fried chicken anymore?"). But if you are determinedly upbeat, secure in the knowledge that you are preparing healthful, tasty meals, chances are good that they'll come around eventually. Teens might do so more readily if some smart rock group would call itself "Low Fat," so that the word would get out via T-shirts, but in the meantime you'll have to do the best you can.

Speaking of teenagers, you might well wonder how you can control what they eat outside the house. It's one thing to stock the refrigerator and cupboard with the "right" foods, but how about when they're out with their friends (read "at the mall")? Well, the simple fact is that some things are out of your control, and this is one of them. Still, just as basic values are instilled at home and are then put into practice by kids out in the big, wide world, this, too, will be an effort you will make at home and hope that some of it rubs off for more permanent use elsewhere. Besides, what you serve at home will help balance the high-fat choices they make on their own, and the daily total of fat consumption will therefore average out more favorably.

Take comfort in the fact that all improvements you make put family members that much ahead of the game, whatever they do on their own. You don't want to be in the position of monitoring everyone's food intake, which would be not only incredibly boring, but also nonproductive in a number of ways, not the least of which would be enormous family friction. There's just so much you yourself can do.

*Getting
the word
out on
Low Fat*

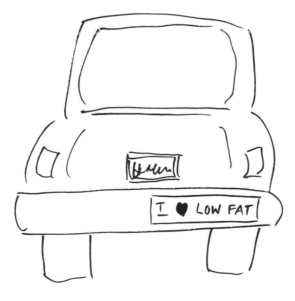

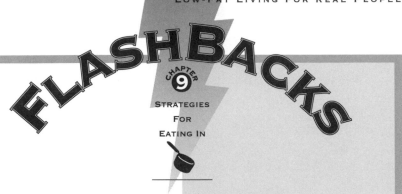

FLASHBACKS

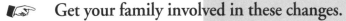

👉 Get your family involved in these changes.

👉 Introduce changes gradually:
- Offer fat-free or 1%-fat milk.
- Reduce fat in dishes you normally prepare.
- Serve an "embarrassingly simple" dish along with the usual fare.

👉 It's okay – a good idea, even – to serve more than one starch and vegetable per meal.

👉 Grill, broil, or poach rather than fry.

👉 Reduce serving sizes of protein foods. (meat/poultry/fish/cheese).

👉 Make sure the food you serve looks attractive and colorful, and that it offers a variety of textures.

👉 Relax and accept that you cannot control what family members eat on their own time.

👉 Remember – you can only do what you can do.

Chapter Ten
Foods Your Heart Will Love

Foods
Your Heart
Will Love

Graduate Level

Congratulations are in order at this point! You've taken the basic course in low-fat living, and, we fervently hope, have a better understanding of The Big Picture. You're already eating plenty of good, healthy foods like fish, beans, starches, fruits, and vegetables. Now we'd like to take you to the Graduate Level, introduce you to some new food concepts, but if you don't feel you're quite ready, hold off for a while. Then come back to this chapter. We'll be waiting for you.

◆　◆　◆　◆

Starches, Fruits, and Vegetables, Revisited

Phytochemicals

Starches, fruits, and vegetables contain thousands of compounds that are not to be confused with vitamins and minerals. They are little "miracle workers," many of which are only now beginning to be studied. While there is still a pleasant mystery to the whole thing, they do have a name: "phytochemicals" (pronounced FIGHT-o-chemicals). We know that plant foods pack a health wallop. They even lower blood pressure.

Who would have thought the nutritional stars of the new millenium would be humble starches, fruits, and vegetables?

Folic Acid

The benefits of eating starches, fruits, and vegetables go beyond merely lowering cholesterol. We all remember when cholesterol was an unfamiliar word, and we know where that went. So it shouldn't surprise you that another new word has come on the scene, and, as luck would have it, another one that would stump the national spelling bee champ. The word is "*homocysteine*" (pronounced homo-SIS-teen), and, like cholesterol, it's circulating in your blood right this minute. Also like cholesterol, it is associated with heart disease.[29]

There are other parallels, too. Homocysteine can be measured in the blood, high homocysteine levels have been found in people with heart disease, and high levels in people without heart disease are at an increased risk of developing the disease.

But there is a big, big difference between these two spelling bee monsters. While cholesterol is old hat at this point, homocysteine is decidedly not. Cholesterol is a mature adult; homocysteine is just a baby, and there is much less hard information available about it. For instance, while it makes sense to lower homocysteine, we don't yet have studies showing that doing so reduces heart disease.

> For great recipes that will help you in your quest for folic acid, try Chickpeas, Fast and Furious, page 155, and Fresh Spinach and Porto-bello Mushrooms, page 166.

But already there's a lot of exciting stuff out there, and the most exciting part of all is that for most people it's really easy to deal with high homocysteine levels. It's even easy to keep them from getting high in the first place. How? With folic acid, a B vitamin found in starchy beans, fruits, and vegetables. (Ah, we hear you say. Now I see why they named this section "Starches, Fruits, and Vegetables, Revisited.")

This is such an important issue that the government has required certain grain products to be "enriched" with folic acid: flour, rice, macaroni, noodles, corn meal, and farina. If your bread, rolls, and buns are being made with "enriched" flour, you're also getting folic acid. And if you're taking a multi-vitamin, you're getting folic acid.[30]

Fiber

Throughout this book we've mentioned FIBER as a good-for-you, heart-protective part of starches, fruits, and vegetables. This is hard to overstate, so we'll re-phrase: People with high-fiber diets have less heart disease. Let's take a closer look.

Foods
Your Heart
Will Love

There are two broad categories of fibers, soluble and insoluble, and some of us spend large parts of the day trying to remember which is which. In fact, "soluble" fiber is, as its name suggests, associated with water, and has Graduate Level names such as pectin, gums, and psyllium. As for insoluble fiber, which has names such as cellulose and hemicellulose, it's the one that "helps promote regularity." Nature's own laxative.

> **BEANS, BEANS...**
>
> 3-6 ounces of cooked starchy beans every day is enough to lower your cholesterol.

The fact is that both are found in most foods with fiber (whole grains, fruits, and vegetables), both are important, and both have a place in the diet. (Both can be also be found in powder and pill form, and in wafers, too, but they are not a replacement for the original packaging—starches, fruits, and vegetables.)

Soluble fiber has traditionally been associated with lowering cholesterol, making it particularly attractive in this day and age. There are a lot of different soluble fibers out there, but here's the kicker: Not all soluble fiber is created equal, and we don't know that they all lower cholesterol. In other words, not everyone can join this club. Club members have demonstrated not only the ability to lower cholesterol, but also how much is needed to get the job done safely. We know that starchy beans and oats are members in good standing.

The big difference between beans and oats is that oatmeal has the necessary studies behind it, so that it is the first that has been allowed by the FDA to make a health claim: "Soluble fiber from oatmeal, as part of a low-saturated fat, low-cholesterol diet, may help reduce the risk of heart disease." (Doesn't exactly have a ring to it, but there you have it.) We're waiting for other studies from other foods for this and other fibers, so that they, too, can make health claims. It's a great big bandwagon, and there are sure to be a host of these claims on foods in years to come.

Keep in mind that it takes money to do those studies, and there are lots of wonderful, healthy foods (we'll mention those starchy beans again) that haven't "unionized," so to speak, so there isn't the necessary money behind them. That is, the fact that they lack a specific health claim does not mean they lack healthy properties.

The First to Have a Health Claim

"The more things change, the more they stay the same," goes the saying, and we're here to tell you that it's certainly true for oatmeal. Grandma ate a hearty bowl of oatmeal for breakfast, and maybe you do, too. The bowl's the same (it may even have been Grandma's), the cereal's the same, but now you've got all kinds of medical research behind your cereal, telling you that it is heart protective. A food your heart will love. Oatmeal has been around for a long time, and now we know it isn't going away.

There are plenty of products out there with oatmeal in them, but not all of them help lower cholesterol (which is why the health claim says "soluble fiber from oatmeal"). In other words, an oatmeal cookie or an oatmeal square or a slice of oatmeal cake just isn't going to do it for you. On the other hand, that cup-and-a-half of oatmeal for breakfast (maybe with fresh fruit on top) is going to do it.

> ## HEADS UP!
>
> How much do you have to eat every day to lower your cholesterol?[31] Ideally, three grams, the amount in one and a half cups of oatmeal or in one cup of oat bran or in three pouches of instant oatmeal. That's a lot of oatmeal, we have to confess, and a hefty portion of oat bran, too, but do what you can. Remember, you're at the Graduate Level now.

There is an essential mystery to food, and often it is the combination of fibers that have beneficial effects. If this statement causes you to wipe your brow in dismay, consider this: all you have to do is eat more whole grains, fruits, and vegetables, which is pretty much what we've been saying all along.

Foods

Your Heart

Will Love

Extra Credit

And so we come to the Extra Credit section, a chance for you to go above and beyond. As is the case with any Extra Credit, it is possible to do well on your exam without doing this, but you just might be better off if you **do** do it. Better off how? Possible protection against cancer and osteoporosis. And lower cholesterol.

Are you ready?

Let's begin with three little letters: S-O-Y. If you've had dealings with it before, it may well have been by adding five other letters: S-A-U-C-E. But there's more to soy than sauce. A lot more. There are heart-protective things found in soy that aren't found anywhere else.

What is soy, anyway? Actually, it starts life as a bean, as in "soybean," and you might even see tender, young soybeans in the freezer section. But that's not the way you generally see soy in the store. You could say that soy is the Master of Disguises, sort of the Lon Chaney of the food world. Like Chaney, it has 1,000 faces (or close to it), and can resemble all kinds of familiar foods. In the grocery store you'll find "tofu," little cheese-like blocks made from soy milk, which you'll also see in the store. In order to get tofu, they separate the curds and whey, and the curds are actually the "cheese." Remember Little Miss Muffet, sitting on her tuffet? Eating her curds and whey? Could be she was a tofu fan, years ahead of her time.

In some circles tofu is extremely popular, and may be used instead of meat in a vegetable stir-fry, for example. The Chinese call tofu "meat without bones," because it has a lot of protein. We call it "chicken without bones," because it sort of looks like it—boneless and skinless.

Speaking of meat, you can find "meats" made from soybeans, "in your grocer's freezer," as the ads used to say—burgers, pork sausages, and pork patties. Green Giant is out there as the first major company with this "faux meat." Morningstar Farms is another brand you can look for. You can go to a health food store and find many more faux meats, freezers full of everything from chicken parmesan to hot dogs, all made from soy. You might consider replacing some of the animal protein in your diet with soy-based food products, an excellent way to cut down on saturated fat ("Mr. Big of the Fats World," if you'll recall). Once you get beyond the world of milk-, cheese-, and meat-like soy foods, you can find a host of completely unfamiliar-looking soy foods in the health food store. No one has even bothered to name them in a familiar way. Consider "miso" and "tempeh" and "natto." They may sound like websites, but they are, we can tell you, real foods, so they might be worth exploring.

So you want to put a little soy in your life? Chances are you've already done so. It is a virtual miracle, and is used in antibiotics, in beer, in printer's ink, and in cosmetics. It's also used in making cardboard, tape joint cements, linoleum backing, putty, soap, and other things too numerous to list here. But we have to mention this: Henry Ford actually envisioned using soybean plastics to build cars.[32]

Now you have a chance to lower cholesterol the soy way. You've come this far, so why not check the very important Endnote[33] to see how much soy you'll need, and what it can do for you. Then you'll need a few letters of introduction, and here they are: ISP. TSP.[34]

SOY FOR THE BEGINNER

ISP: soy powder. How to use it? Try making a milkshake with fat-free milk, a little Hershey's syrup, a ripe banana, and 1/4 cup of ISP.

TSP: soy stuffing. How to use it? Go to the grocery store and buy a faux meat.

Tofu: How to use it? Get a good tofu cookbook, such as *Tofu Cookery* by Louise Hagler (Book Publishing Company).

Soy milk: How to use it? Drink it. Check the supermarket for various brands and try them to see which you like best. Our personal favorite, however, requires a trip to the health food store: Westbrae Natural health drinks, specifically WestSoy Lite Malted Nondairy Drink. It comes in a nifty little no-glass-to-wash package, with its own cute straw attached.

Miso: How to use it? Add a tablespoon to your soups, sauces, and gravies for added flavor.

Okay, now you know something about soy. If you want to know more, there's actually an 800 number you can call, and we'll bet you can guess what it is, even if we don't tell you. But we will: (800) TALK SOY.

Garlic

Our grandmothers used to tell us that if you ate lots of garlic, you would never get sick. We told Grandma that if you didn't get sick, it was because anyone who was already sick would refuse to come close enough to pass the germs on to you, thanks to all that garlic you were eating. Now it seems Grandma might have had a point.

We know that garlic tastes great—cooked with onions and tomatoes, for instance, and poured over pasta—but now it turns out that there may, just may, be actual health benefits associated with eating it. Might be worth getting some into your food every day. Garlic has its own special language. Fresh garlic comes as a "head," which sort of looks like an onion that has lots of little segments. Each of these segments is called a "clove," not to be confused with cloves, the spicy spice that gives pumpkin pie, say, its kick. Each garlic clove comes in something that looks like a tissue-paper wrapper, which you take off before using the garlic. This is less tedious if you imagine you are opening tiny birthday presents. Or you can buy a labor-saving device specifically made for the job that is nothing more than a rubber tube. Stick a few cloves inside the tube and roll them around with your palm; the tissue-like skin peels itself right off. Caution: This is actually kind of fun, and you may find yourself with a lot more peeled garlic than the one to three cloves you're looking for.[35]

Nuts

If you like anagrams, those word games in which letters in a word are switched around to make another word, consider "N-U-T-S." The same letters spell "STUN," and you may be stunned to discover that nuts are good for you.

But, you may ask, aren't nuts high in fat? The answer is yes, but nuts are a "Better Bet" as a fat. The also contain folic acid, fiber, and Vitamin

E. Your heart will love them. Studies show that people who eat nuts have less heart disease than those who do not.[36]

We're not (sorry about this) telling you to work your way through a jar of nuts and call it dinner. We are urging you to use nuts regularly, but use them as a garnish. You can see (at right) how much fat you're getting when you use nuts, so don't go overboard.

> **ONE TEASPOON OF FAT IS EQUAL TO:**
>
> 6 almonds
> 3 jumbo cashews
> 10 peanuts (large),
>   or 2 teaspoons
>   peanut butter
> 4 pecan halves
> 18 pistachios
> 4 walnut halves

Foods

Your Heart

Will Love

Vitamin E

Now here's a paradox worthy of Graduate Level discussion. Vitamin E, most commonly found in foods high in fat, seems to be heart protective. Obviously if you reduce the fat in your diet, you are also reducing the amount of vitamin E. If you don't reduce the fat, you have another set of problems, and that's what this whole book is about, isn't it? The truth is you can't get enough vitamin E from food alone, even on a high-fat diet, so see if your doctor recommends a vitamin E supplement. It may not exactly be "a food your heart will love," but there's a good chance your heart will love it anyway.

LDL

At the Graduate Level you can, of course, expect to be graded, so think of your LDL level (that's the "lousy" cholesterol) as your grade. Just remember that you want a low score, not a high one—like golf.

By lowering your cholesterol level in general, you are specifically trying to get the LDL down, and we've shown you some interesting food-related ways to do that. Obviously you want to reduce your risk of heart disease as much as you possibly can.

If you already have heart disease, you'd like to put yourself in the best

Your goal is to lower your LDL (the "lousy" cholesterol).

Foods

Your Heart

Will Love

possible position to bring it under control.

Sometimes, though, no matter what you do it isn't enough. You eat well, maybe even at the Graduate Level, you exercise (and we do want you to exercise), but you still may have an unacceptably high LDL level. Remember that it is only partly under your control, since your body manufactures two-thirds of the cholesterol in your blood. In other words, changing your diet (and exercising) may not do the trick for you.

The good news is that we live in a pleasantly high-tech era, and there are medications available that can help. Do form a partnership with your doctor. If you're old enough to remember listening to the Top Ten on your 45's, you're definitely ready for that partnership. It's the best present you can give yourself. Think of it as a birthday present, because we want you to have a lot of birthdays. In fact, it's why we wrote this book.

Chapter Eleven
Frequently Asked Questions –and the Answers

CHAPTER

Frequently
Asked
Questions
– and the
Answers

?

Frequently

Asked

Questions

— and the

Answers

If these questions speak to you, you have a lot of company. They are questions that we've been asked (professionally and nonprofessionally) over and over again.

Q: Am I eating low fat if I buy only foods that say "Low Cholesterol"?

A: Not necessarily. You have to check the food label for total fat. Low cholesterol and low fat are not the same thing.[37]

Q: Am I eating low cholesterol if I eat foods that are low in fat?

A: Most likely. Foods that are low in fat tend to be low in cholesterol, with the exception of organ meats (brains, liver, kidneys).

Q: Isn't margarine better than butter?

A: The jury is still out on that one. Meanwhile, we **do** know that less is better.

Q: How about diet margarine?

A: Diet margarine is simply regular margarine with air beaten into it, meaning there is less fat in a serving, and less fat is better. If you can stand the taste.

Q: Not to push this margarine thing, but what am I supposed to use on my toast in the morning?

A: We don't know you personally, but are you someone with the discipline to use just a smidgin (the "scientific" term for half a teaspoon)? That translates into one stick of butter seeing you through 48 breakfasts! If your stick disappears in a week, try jam, jelly, marmalade, or honey on your toast. They contain no fat at all.

Q: Are you suggesting I fry with jam or jelly?

A: No, we're suggesting that you don't fry at all! Nonstick skillets are wonderful, and if you still need a bit of fat, use spray oil, which you can get in the supermarket. But use it sparingly.

Q: What about fat-free mayonnaise, cream cheese, sour cream, and all that?

A: When you decide to go easy on fat, these are great to begin with, assuming you don't mind the loss of taste (less apparent when you are combining a number of ingredients in a recipe). And these products offer the comfort of the familiar without the fat. However, there are new and wonderful tastes out there, tastes that go beyond the creaminess of mayonnaise and sour cream, and you'll want to try them. Check out the recipes in the back of this book (beginning on page 137).

Q: In order to eat "low fat," do I have to eat vegetarian?

A: No, no, no, no, no! Absolutely not!

Still, if only for the sake of variety, it's kind of nice to eat vegetarian every once in a while (pasta's always good), but remember that vegetarian dishes are not necessarily low in fat. Again, the recipes in the back of this book will give you lots of ideas.

Q: I've heard that bananas are fatty. Is that true?

A: No. Bananas don't contain fat. Fruits, as well as vegetables, are as close as you can get to no-fat foods. There are a few fatty exceptions, such as avocados and olives, and you simply have to go easy on these.

As far as gaining weight goes, you'd have to eat an awful lot of bananas to gain weight. How many overweight monkeys have you seen lately?

Q: Can I eat nuts on a low-fat diet?

A: Yes, only think of them as garnishes. They contain a lot of fat, but it's a "good" fat – monounsaturated. Interesting bit of trivia: Chestnuts, despite their name, contain very little fat.

Q: What do I do about salt on a low-fat diet?

A: Naturally your body is happier without too much salt, but low-fat eating is a separate issue. In other words, you don't have to eat less salt on a low-fat diet.

Q: How about sugar? If I eat low sugar, will I be eating low fat?

A: Probably not. While it's true that lots of sugary foods also contain a whole lot of fat (ice cream, baked goods, et cetera), sugar and fat are not the same thing. Eating less sugar doesn't mean you are also eating less fat. Besides, if you eat many sugary foods, you won't be eating all the "good stuff" (okay, okay, we all have our own definition of "good stuff") like fruits and vegetables, which really are low in fat.

Q: Can't I just take a vitamin instead of lowering the fat in my diet?

A: There is no substitute for a low-fat diet. Vitamins can't make fat go away. Maybe you've heard people say, "I wish there was a magic pill for this." We all do. And we're still looking for one.

Q: What about fat-free cakes and cookies?

A: Ah, you mean Fat-Free Chocolate-Covered Creme-Filled Mini-Cakes. They are popular, all right, and we suppose they're an option if eaten occasionally and in intelligent serving sizes. They have no nutritional value, though. And they have plenty of calories. Fat free doesn't mean calorie free.

Q: What's with these food labels? They look like a math test I forgot to study for! I'm trying to figure out how much fat I'm getting, and I don't know where to look first.

A: It's really not all that complicated. Just take a look at serving size, because everything on the label is based on one serving of that food. Then look at "Total Fat." By the way, if there are 3 grams or less, you are looking at a low-fat food – assuming you eat the same size serving as the one listed on the package.

Q: But my serving size is bigger than the one on the label!

A: Then you're getting more fat than you think you are. Remember that even a low-fat food may no longer be low fat if you eat a lot of it.

Q: I'm on a low-fat diet, but I'm getting rounder and rounder! How is that possible?

A: Either your OPSS (Own Personal Serving Size) for your food in general is too big, or you aren't moving around enough.

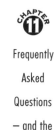

Q: What about exercise?

A: If you are asking this question in the first place, most likely you are not doing a hard, 30-minute workout three or four times a week. But there is another way to work out. Would you believe leaf raking, housework, and brisk walking are all considered exercise? Put them all together for 30 minutes every day. The good news is that you don't have to do the entire 30 minutes at once; try three ten-minute spurts of activity.

Q: I'm sick and tired of chicken! Is there anything else I can eat instead?

A: Sounds like you're in a "chicken rut." Food is like a theme park. Obviously you don't always want to take the same ride. So try other rides! See the next question.

Q: Can I eat beef? Pork?

A: Yes, but not all the time, maybe once or twice a week. Check labels for "Extra Lean" or "Lean," preferably the former, which is lower in fat. Remember to think "deck of cards," not "placemat," when it comes to serving size.

Q: Can I eat shrimp?

A: Yes, and ignore those who make comments about the cholesterol it contains. Again, don't eat it all the time, and pay attention to that 3-ounce serving size. If you buy 6 ounces of raw shrimp in the shell, you will have 3 ounces of cooked shrimp at home.[38]

Q: Should I avoid fatty fish?

A: No. All fish is good for you, and the fat in fish is not the kind of fat you have to worry about. The only kind of "fatty fish" you want to stay away from is the kind that comes deep fried.

Q: I hate this. How about if I just eat "Healthy Choice" for lunch and dinner every day?

A: You're going to get very, very bored. After a while everything will begin to taste the same, and you'll get sick of the whole thing and give up even the pretense of eating low fat. The trick is to commit yourself to finding new foods that taste good and are easy to prepare. Which is, after all, one reason why you bought this book, isn't it?

Q: I like to eat pizza on Friday nights. Any suggestions?

A: We assume you want to continue this tradition, so why not make the pizza as low in fat as possible? While you're at it, go out with like-minded friends so you can order one pizza with extra vegetables instead of the usual (high in fat) pepperoni or sausage. Then ask for half the cheese. In fact, many places now make delicious no-cheese pizzas. Finally, have a salad and extra bread so two slices will satisfy you.

Q: What's the deal with olive oil? I see "light," "virgin," "extra virgin" in the supermarket. Which is better?

A: Olive oil is olive oil, really. The difference is flavor. If you don't like a strong taste, choose "light." As to "virgin" and "extra virgin," we prefer the latter, because we like it as a concept.

Q: It's holiday time! I look forward to this all year! Are you suggesting I give up my traditional holiday treats?

A: Of course not. Eat and enjoy. We are, however, suggesting that you not *over*eat. When you really, truly binge, you feel really, truly terrible anyway, and there you are popping antacid tablets (admittedly fat free). But if you just go easy, even though you may be eating high-fat foods, you won't be eating so much of them, which will automatically mean lower fat. Also, you might want to introduce one low-fat dish to the holiday table – maybe Pumpkin Pie-less, a pumpkin custard (see recipe, page 226).

Q: What if I crave chocolate, which I know is high in fat?

A: Go for fat free! Use Hershey's syrup. Eat a fat-free Fudgsicle. Or get yourself a small chocolate bar, preferably dark chocolate, which appears to be less damaging to the heart. Better than buying the extraordinarily large, pass-around size that you'll eat all by yourself anyhow. By the way, if you buy the most expensive chocolate bar you can find, you'll be less likely to get the large size.

Q: I love good ice cream. I've tried that fat-free frozen yogurt, but it's a pretty bad substitute. Any ideas?

A: Check out various brands of fat-free frozen yogurt. Some are, we admit, not much in the flavor department, but others are very good. Taste being the individual issue that it is, you'll want to "taste test" for yourself. If all else fails, you're better off with a small amount of low-fat frozen yogurt rather than going back to premium ice cream. If you are buying a cup of frozen yogurt at the mall, say, Colombo's is a good fat-free choice. If you are standing in the freezer section at the supermarket, remember to read labels. Many frozen yogurts are quite high in fat. Breyer's is an example of one that is low in fat; Dannon and Sealtest Free are fat free.

Q: I've checked the Ingredient List on my bread and pasta, just like you want me to do, and I see there is no added fat. So how come the Nutrition Facts label tells me there is 1 gram of fat?

A: Small amounts of fat occur naturally in grains. Don't worry about it.

Q: I stopped off for fries after work yesterday. Guess I shouldn't have done that, huh?

A: What does "should" or "shouldn't" have to do with it? The fact that you "stopped off for fries" means only one thing. You ate fries. We suggest you not do this often, but we certainly hope they were good, and that you really enjoyed them!

Q: I'm afraid to cook low fat for guests. Or even in-laws, for that matter. What if the food doesn't taste good?

A: We'll hope it's better next time. Meanwhile, you've given it a good shot. Keep up the good work. After all, you are protecting your family and yourself. Your guests, too, as a matter of fact.

Q: I don't know where to start with this low-fat business!

A: Do something, anything, so you'll know you can start, that you can

Frequently

Asked

Questions

– and the

Answers

do it. We suggest putting some cut-up fruit in your salad, maybe pear or cantaloupe. Tonight.

Q: Yes, but I don't have time to cut up fruit.

A: No problem. Every grocery store sells cut-up fruit.

Q: Yes, but what if my family doesn't like fruit in the salad?

A: How do you know if you don't try? This low-fat stuff takes day-to-day persistence. You'll be trying lots of new things.

Q: Yes, but I don't want to try new things! Too much work!

A: We notice a pattern here. All your questions begin with "yes, but." Sounds like you're not really convinced about this. It's your own personal rebellion.

Q: I'm afraid I did something wrong, something that caused my spouse's heart disease!

A: Relax. There are many things that contribute to heart disease. The real question is: Now what? How can I protect my family? Re-read this book to find out exactly what you can do.

Q: My kids and my spouse eat low fat at home, but as soon as they leave the house, it's another story. What can I do about that?

A: Not much. You have obviously set an example at home, and that's about all you can do.

Q: My spouse will not eat low fat. What can I do about *that*?

A: We assume you're doing the cooking, which means that you are probably not cooking the same way you used to. You might try making some of the old favorites from time to time, and negotiating the rest.

And give yourself time – months, maybe many months. This doesn't have to happen overnight. Remember that anything you can do to reduce fat in the diet is helpful, and that even the smallest step is a step in the right direction.

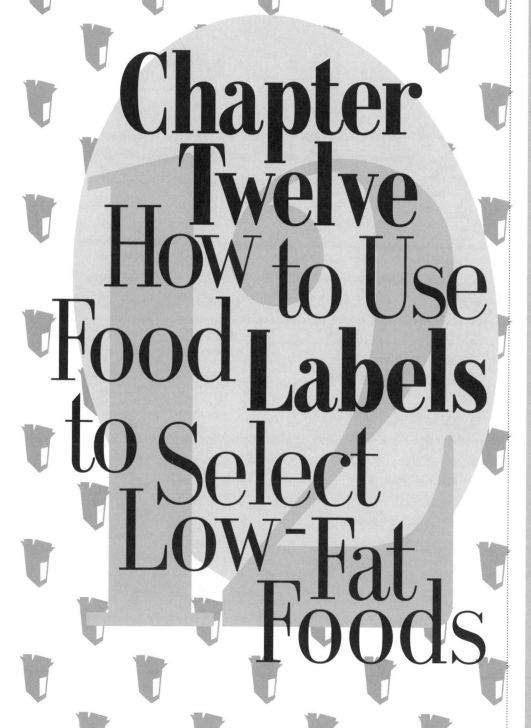

Chapter Twelve
How to Use Food Labels to Select Low-Fat Foods

How to Use

Food Labels

to Select

Low-Fat Foods

Understanding the Food Label

We've been talking a lot about choosing foods that are low in fat – the kinds of meats, the kinds of starches, the kinds of snacks that fit into a low-fat diet. We've seen that what you assume to be low in fat may not be if you eat a whole lot of it.

Labels give you a shot at figuring out how much fat is actually in the foods you buy. Unfortunately, not all foods are required to have labels. If they are too small, like Vienna sausages, or the companies are too small, like Uncle John's Magic Morning Tofu Drink, or if the food is a raw food,[39] or is located in the bakery or the delicatessen section, it doesn't have to have a label. Check the Endnote[40] for information on fat content in your favorite deli foods. Be prepared to have your socks knocked off. But keep in mind that label free doesn't mean fat free. If there is no sign next to those tempting muffins the size of headlight bulbs, you might try the "napkin test," which involves setting a muffin on a paper napkin, then taking it off and looking for a telltale grease spot. Too bad that, by the time you see the spot, you are already the proud owner of a fat-laden muffin.

READ LABELS!

That's where all the information is.

With no nutrition information required on breads, rolls, and cakes, on freshly sliced lunch meats and cheeses, on prepared salads and appetizers, on desserts – well, let's just say they aren't making things easy for us, are they?

Take a look at the label.

Nutrition Facts		
Serving Size 1 cup (228g)		
Servings Per Container 2		
Amount Per Serving		
Calories 260 Calories from Fat 120		
		% Daily Value*
Total Fat 13g		**20%**
Saturated Fat 5g		**25%**
Cholesterol 30mg		**10%**
Sodium 660mg		**28%**
Total Carbohydrate 31g		**10%**
Dietary Fiber 0g		**0%**
Sugars 5g		
Protein 5g		
Vitamin A 4% • Vitamin C 2%		
Calcium 15% • Iron 4%		

* Percent Daily Values are based on a 2,000 calorie diet. Your daily values may be higher or lower depending on your calorie needs.

		Calories:	2,000	2,500
Total Fat	Less than		65g	80g
Sat Fat	Less than		20g	25g
Cholesterol	Less than		300mg	300mg
Sodium	Less than		2,400mg	2,400mg
Total Carbohydrate			300g	375g
Dietary Fiber			25g	30g

Calories per gram:
Fat 9 • Carbohydrate 4 • Protein 4

Serving Size

At the top of the label is serving size, and the big news here is that *Serving Size is the most important item on the label, because everything that follows is based on that.* Understand this is the amount commonly consumed. It is not a recommended amount.

Besides, the serving size doesn't necessarily bear much resemblance to the amount you, personally, eat. As we've encouraged you to do throughout this book, think OPSS (Own Personal Serving Size) when reading a label. How big is your serving? Compare it to the amount on the label and you may find that you have some calculating to do. (Remember, it doesn't take much to go from OPSS to OOPS!) It makes no difference what the label calls "one serving"; if you eat two or three times that, then everything else on the label, grams of fat included, will have to be multiplied by two or three or whatever.

◆   ◆   ◆   ◆

Let's take a look at that label again. Because there are so many facts, let's narrow our focus, and we'll bet you can guess where the focus will be, namely, on label information for Total Fat and Saturated Fat. (If you're wondering why not Cholesterol, we'll say once again: A diet low in fat will also be low in cholesterol, unless you are eating organ meats – brains, liver, kidneys.)

Nutrition Facts	
Serving Size 1 cup (228g)	
Servings Per Container 2	
Amount Per Serving	
Calories 260 Calories from Fat 120	
	% Daily Value
Total Fat 13g	20%
Saturated Fat 5g	25%
Cholesterol 30mg	10%
Sodium 660mg	28%
Total Carbohydrate 31g	10%
Dietary Fiber 0g	0%
Sugars 5g	
Protein 5g	

Grams

As you look at this label, you can see that Nutrition Facts about Total Fat and Saturated Fat are presented in two ways. One, which has been around for a long time, simply gives the grams of fat in a serving of the food. (As we've seen earlier in this book, a gram is a unit of weight, about that of a straight pin.) You can consider the product is low in Total Fat if it contains no more than 3 grams of fat in one serving. As for Saturated Fat – it's so incredibly undesirable that to be considered low Saturated Fat, a serving of food may contain no more than 1 gram of that fat.

So much for grams. The other way in which fat information is presented is Percent Daily Value.

Percent Daily Value

Hold on tight, now. This isn't easy to understand, so read S-L-O-W-L-Y.

Percent Daily Value for fat is the relationship between the amount of fat in a serving of that product and the total amount of fat you might reasonably eat in a day (Daily Value). The Percent Daily Value for fat can be used as a screening mechanism that tells you at a glance whether there's a lot or a little fat in the particular product, and therefore whether or not you should even consider buying it. **So look for foods that have:**

5% OR LESS DAILY VALUE FOR TOTAL FAT

The Nutrition Labeling and Education Act has given specific guidelines for "low" Total Fat, Saturated Fat, Cholesterol, and Sodium. The figures are given in metric measurements, which is to say grams and milligrams.

By taking the value for "low" and dividing by the Daily Value, we get 5%. Take Total Fat for example:

$$\frac{3 \text{ grams}}{65 \text{ grams}} \; = \; 5\%$$

You can do the math for Saturated Fat, Cholesterol, and Sodium. The result will be the same – or something close to it.

Looking Back At — And Beyond — The Label

A certain number of a day's calories can come from fat, but not too many, no more than 30 percent of the total number of calories you take in each day.   Considering that this figure is 35-40 percent for the average American,[41] 30 percent is a significant improvement. But some studies have shown that even 30 percent isn't low enough. A therapeutic reduced-fat diet may be closer to 10 percent fat and has, in fact, been shown by Dr. Dean Ornish to reverse heart disease – that is, clear the arteries.[42]

The Ornish study included other significant lifestyle changes as well, such as daily meditation, three hours of exercise per week, and weekly group therapy sessions. Following such a regimen was difficult but rewarding for participants and those who cared about them. (This diet is not for everyone, however, and should not be followed without professional guidance.)

Whether you are following a 10 percent fat diet (exceedingly difficult), a 30 percent fat diet (undoubtedly a happy change from your old habits), or something in between (good for you!), you can use labels as a tool. Maybe it's an imperfect one, but it can remind you of how much fat you take in each day.

If you like to keep careful track of such things, you can use the food labels to *tally grams of fat*. Easier than scoring bowling or bridge.

Or you can *use percentages*. You can tell by the bold typeface that the folks responsible for the food labels (the FDA) are putting a lot of weight behind them. We've seen their usefulness (Percent Daily Value) as a screening tool to choose foods low in Total Fat and Saturated Fat, and how the magic 5% quickly identifies these foods.

But life is never perfect, and this is no exception. While labels can tell you whether or not a particular food is low in fat, for example, they can only do so much. Besides, a lot of the food you eat doesn't come in bags

How to Use

Food Labels

to Select

Low-Fat Foods

or boxes or any other package. You cook, you eat out, you live a life that is largely label free.

Eventually, true knowledge will take over. You won't have to calculate grams of fat, or Percent Daily Value, or anything else, because you will have become so familiar with how things fit together that you will understand the relative place of fat in the diet. You'll know, for example, that there are more and more low-fat and fat-free foods on the market every day. You'll know which cuts of meat are lowest in fat, and that you don't need to eat much of them. You'll know that you'll do better if you avoid cream-based soups, sauces, and gravies, and anything deep fried. An appealing fringe benefit will be that you'll actually feel better when there is less fat in your diet, and you'll very likely come to the point where you find thick, fatty foods unappealing. Tastes do change. When you were a kid, you hated (What? Soup? Potatoes? Vegetables?) and now you're known throughout your zip code for your fabulous minestrone.

Give yourself a chance. It's worth it.

Chapter Thirteen
Embarrassingly Simple Recipes

CHAPTER
13

Embarrassingly

Simple

Recipes

How To Avoid "White Knuckle" Cooking

"White knuckle" cooking is familiar to you if you are excessively concerned with recipe directions, if you cannot imagine cooking anything when the measuring spoons or measuring cup are in the dishwasher. Fear and/or panic leads to a death-grip on the spatula, and your knuckles turn white.

We hope you will relax a little bit, because, although this may be a funny thing to say in a book containing recipes, don't worry too much about following these recipes exactly. Even when they are very, very specific ("4 teaspoons mustard"), that's really only an estimate of how much of a certain ingredient you might like to use. Four teaspoons could be too much, or not enough, or, as Goldilocks may have discovered, just right. To a great extent the amount of garlic, for instance, that you use depends on how much you feel like chopping. So don't be afraid to vary recipes to suit your own taste. On the other hand, if you come upon a recipe for, say, chicken with apricot jam, and you happen to detest apricots, either try another kind of jam or look for another recipe.

These recipes are all embarrassingly simple. None is simply embarrassing. Some of them hardly deserve to be called recipes at all, but what the heck, we'll call them recipes anyway. They are as close as we could get to what one woman said she was looking for: "Recipes that don't have 'ingredients.'" They take so little time to make that they are actually faster than take-out.

Easy recipes are important, because dinner time has a way of coming around night after night, and sometimes you feel just plain unprepared. Here's a tip: When it's getting to be that time, just begin to sauté some onions. The odor will fill the house and everyone will think Big Things are happening in the kitchen. This will buy you the time you need to figure out what in the world to make for dinner – which may or may not have anything to do with onions.

◆   ◆   ◆   ◆

"**E**mbarrassingly simple" is only half the story. In order to be low fat, recipes follow certain rules, which you'll be applying to recipes wherever you find them. Put these rules together and you wind up with food that is low in total fat as well as saturated fat and cholesterol:

- Servings are held to 3 ounces of Extra Lean meat, fish, or poultry.
- If dairy products are used, they are fat free or low fat.
- If fat is added, it is monounsaturated (olive or canola oil).
- Added fat is held to one teaspoon per serving. This rule may be broken for real salad dressing (see recipe for Our Favorite Oil and Vinegar Dressing, page 189) or for an occasional real treat (see recipe for Vanilla Soufflé to Remember, page 228), but always with an eye on The Big Picture.

Nutrient analysis is a standard part of recipes nowadays, and we have included the calories, fat, carbohydrate, protein, and sodium per serving in each recipe given here. Because these are heart-healthy recipes, the nutrient levels stay within the guidelines suggested by the label law.[43] And we have provided "sodium alerts" for those on sodium-restricted diets.

You'll notice these recipes make use of special flavor enhancers – broth, wine, yogurt, mustard, tomatoes, and fruit. We don't want low fat to be synonymous with low flavor.

You'll notice several soups are included. You might not consider making your own soup to be embarrassingly simple, but if you just add salad, bread, and fruit, you have a nice, light meal, and that makes them very convenient. (Imagine – making your own soup and finding that you've actually saved time!) We prefer to think of them as "floating casseroles." Like ordinary casseroles, they can be made ahead and reheated when needed.

CHAPTER **13**

Embarrassingly
Simple
Recipes

*Low fat
doesn't have
to mean low
flavor.*

SODIUM ALERT!

If you are on a sodium-restricted diet, then use, for example, Health Valley "no salt added" chicken broth.

And you'll notice there are no meat recipes. You've been cooking embarrassingly simple meat recipes for years (also known as throwing hamburgers on the grill), and you don't need to hear more about that here. Besides, as we have noted before, people have chosen chicken as a kind of "transition food" in an effort to eat low fat. We therefore offer chicken recipes, fish recipes, plus quite a number of main dishes that contain neither chicken nor fish.

No-Fat Flavor Enhancers

CHICKEN BROTH: Chicken broth is an embarrassingly simple, no-fat (*assuming you take the fat off*) flavor enhancer. The down-side is that the convenient canned versions tend to be high in salt, but the upside is that there are lower salt versions available as well.

> **BEST HOT TIP OF THE DECADE AND WELL WORTH REPEATING:**
>
> Unless it's fat free, store canned chicken broth in the refrigerator. All the fat will congeal on top, just begging to be removed in an unattractive lump and thrown away.

VEGETABLE BROTH: Swanson makes a canned, clear vegetable broth, and College Inn makes a red one. The broth is very, very low in fat (but high in salt, so a little goes a long way) and is full of flavor. And if the food you cook has a lot of flavor, you won't miss the fat you've eliminated.

WINE: It provides excellent, no-fat flavor, with most (but not all) of the alcohol evaporating during cooking. And how's this for a "seal of approval"? Wine is used in more than a few of the recipes in *The American Heart Association Low-Fat, Low-Cholesterol Cookbook*.

YOGURT: Ah, cream, the basis for many fine, rich foods – and heart disease. For a creamy texture without a medical alert, use fat-free yogurt. It is a chameleon that, seasoned with herbs and spices, or with mustard added, becomes a flavorful marinade, dip, or dressing.

MUSTARD: There are many tasty mustards in the supermarket, and you'll find them made, for example, with wine, dill, honey, and champagne. Experiment with them in your salad dressings. Mustard is delicious spread on fish or chicken before cooking, and is a nice, fat-free addition to tuna or salmon salad. (By the way, check labels and pick a mustard with no fat in it. In particular, mustards with horseradish, or that call themselves "creamy," tend to contain fat.)

> **TO THICKEN YOGURT:**
>
> Put a coffee filter in a strainer, then put the strainer over a bowl. Fill strainer with plain, fat-free yogurt. Cover and put the whole thing in the refrigerator. The longer you leave it there, the thicker the yogurt will get. Twenty minutes will see some results, but if you leave it for several hours or overnight, you'll be left with yogurt that is thick and cream cheese-like. Mixed with a little mustard, it is wonderful to use on sandwiches instead of mayonnaise.

TOMATOES: All sorts of tomato products enhance flavors wonderfully and you'll find that a number of the following recipes make use of tomatoes. Those calling for tomato sauce or crushed tomatoes manage to deliver a lot of sodium along with flavor, so if you are cutting back on sodium, look for low-sodium versions in the supermarket. (Low-sodium alternative brands are suggested along with the recipes.) Fresh and sun-dried tomatoes are not high in sodium.

FRUIT: Fruit juices, preserves, and just plain fruit add remarkable flavor to all sorts of dishes. (You've been using lemon juice right along, probably not even thinking of it as a fruit juice. But it is.) Fruit juice can be used as a marinade or a cooking liquid, preserves can be spread on poultry, for example, before cooking, and fruit can be added to salads. And when there is fruit in the salad, less dressing is needed, an added advantage.

Embarrassingly

Simple

Recipes

Making Food Juicy Without Fat

MARINATING: By soaking food in something before you cook it, you make it juicier, tastier, and more tender. Plain, fat-free yogurt can be flavored with herbs and spices or mustard, thus miraculously becoming a fat-free marinade. So does fat-free salad dressing, available in every supermarket. (Choose low-sodium versions if you are restricting sodium.) Wine, which is fat free, makes a fine marinade, too.

All marinating has in common the fact that the process goes on without you. Just get things going in the morning, even the night before, and when it comes time to do the cooking, great things will have happened in your absence.

USING FOIL: You can make foods juicy by adding liquid – broth, wine, or crushed tomatoes in juice, for example – and sealing with foil. Foil allows food to steam in the flavorful juices. It also makes cleanup embarrassingly simple, since it pretty much comes down to "crumple and toss."

◆   ◆   ◆   ◆

O ccasionally you may want to use just a bit of fat in your cooking, in which case you can *sauté*. High heat makes a *small amount of fat* in the pan go a long way. Sauté means "jump" in French, and you don't need much fat to make that happen. In fact, you can buy cooking oil in a spray can, then spray a very, very light coating in a nonstick skillet (just a puff, really), and get away with a whole lot less fat. This fast cooking gives foods – sliced mushrooms, say – an entirely different (and delicious) flavor.

Here we go. The "star-studded recipes."

Rice, Pasta, Potatoes, Barley, and Beans

> STARCHES? THEY'RE STARTING WITH STARCHES?

The order of recipes may at first seem unfamiliar, but actually it follows the Pyramid. That is, we've stressed starches and vegetables early on, because that's what we'd like you to stress as you plan your meals.

Embarrassingly

Simple

Recipes

Rice, Pasta, and Spinach — Together at Last
4 Servings

In this recipe you want to brown the rice and spaghetti before they start to cook. As you can see, when you use a nonstick skillet you need very little oil. (In fact, you can often get away with none at all.)

If you prefer, you can make this without the spinach. We know a nine-year-old who won't eat much of anything but loves the spinach-free version.

> **1 teaspoon olive oil**
> **1 medium onion, chopped**
> **3/4 cup uncooked rice**
> **1/4 cup uncooked thin spaghetti, broken in 1-inch pieces**
> **1 14-ounce can (approx.) fat-free, lower-sodium chicken broth**
> **3/4 cup water**
> **1 package frozen spinach, thawed and drained (to thaw, run under cold water)**

Using a large, nonstick skillet, heat the oil and cook onion until transparent. Add rice and pasta. Stir until lightly browned. Add broth and water and bring to a boil. Reduce heat, cover with lid or foil, and cook for 15 minutes. Stir in spinach with fork, cover again, and cook until liquid is absorbed, about 15 minutes more.

Per Serving:
Calories: 148 **Fat:** 2g **Carbohydrate:** 26g
Protein: 7g   **Sodium:** 395mg

> **SODIUM ALERT!**
>
> If you are on a sodium-restricted diet, then use, for example, Health Valley "no salt added" chicken broth.

Embarrassingly

Simple

Recipes

Barley and Tomatoes with Apples

(if you can imagine)

4 Servings

If you've never used barley before, you'll find it in the supermarket with the rice and dried beans. It comes in a box or a plastic bag, your choice.

1 28-ounce can tomatoes, drained and chopped

1 14-ounce can (approx.) fat-free, lower-sodium chicken broth

1 ¼ cups water

1 cup barley

1 medium onion, chopped

3 medium Granny Smith apples, peeled, cored, and sliced thin, about 2 cups

Put tomatoes, broth, and water in a large saucepan. Bring to a boil. Add barley and chopped onion, reduce heat, cover, and cook for 30 minutes. Add apples. Cook another 15 minutes, until liquid is absorbed.

Per Serving:

Calories: 205   **Fat:** 1g   **Carbohydrate:** 46g
Protein: 3g   **Sodium:** 660mg

> **SODIUM ALERT!**
>
> If you are on a sodium-restricted diet, then use, for example, Eden "no salt added" canned tomatoes, and Health Valley "no salt added" chicken broth.

Embarrassingly

Simple

Recipes

Not-Too-Boring Potato-Onion Casserole
4 Servings

Not only does this recipe have no added fat, but, because it's a casserole, it can be prepared ahead and cooked at dinner time.

> **4 medium Idaho potatoes**
> **2 medium onions**
> **1 teaspoon dried basil**
> **1 teaspoon dried, crushed bay leaf**
> **1 14-ounce can (approx.) fat-free, lower-sodium chicken broth**
> **Dried herb seasoning**

Preheat oven to 400°F.

Peel potatoes and slice thin. Put in cold water. Cut onions in thin slices. Using a shallow baking dish that can be placed on the stovetop, layer potatoes, onions, basil, and bay leaf. Continue to layer until used up.

Pour chicken broth over the top. Sprinkle with herb seasoning. Bring to a boil on the stove, cover with foil, reduce heat, and simmer for 5 minutes. Put in oven and bake, uncovered, for 25 minutes.

Per Serving:
Calories: 137 **Fat:** 1g **Carbohydrate:** 28g
Protein: 4g   **Sodium:** 275mg

SODIUM ALERT!

If you are on a sodium-restricted diet, then use, for example, Health Valley "no salt added" chicken broth.

Potatoes Foil-Roasted on the Grill

4 Servings

Embarrassingly

Simple

Recipes

1 ½ pounds red-skinned potatoes, cubed (do not peel)
Dried herb seasoning
Garlic powder
Nonstick cooking spray
Heavy aluminum foil, large enough to make an envelope
around the potatoes

Spread the potatoes evenly on the foil, sprinkle with herb seasoning and garlic powder, then spray LIGHTLY with oil. Place packet on charcoal grill and cook for 30 minutes, turning once after 10 minutes and again after 20 minutes.

Per Serving:
Calories: 113   **Fat:** 0g   **Carbohydrate:** 2g   **Protein:** 3g   **Sodium:** 28g

Embarrassingly

Simple

Recipes

Red-Hot Roasted Potatoes
4 Servings

Actually, these are medium hot. If you really like the feeling of fire in your mouth, experiment with adding more chili powder and cayenne pepper—at your own risk!

> **Nonstick cooking spray**
> **1/4 cup Dijon mustard**
> **1/2 teaspoon chili powder**
> **1/8 teaspoon cayenne pepper**
> **1 tablespoon lemon juice**
> **16 small red potatoes, cut in half**

Preheat oven to 400°F.

Spray roasting pan lightly with cooking spray. (For easy cleanup, first line pan with foil.) Put mustard, chili powder, cayenne pepper, and lemon juice in a medium bowl. Mix together, then add potatoes and toss well to coat them with the mixture. Put into roasting pan in single layer, keeping them from touching. Bake 45 minutes to 1 hour, turning once, until tender. Serve hot or at room temperature.

Per Serving:
Calories: 113   **Fat:** 0g   **Carbohydrate:** 30g   **Protein:** 4g   **Sodium:** 0mg

Sweet Potato "Chips"

4 Servings

This is a taste treat that is easy to prepare because you don't have to peel the potatoes.

2 large unpeeled, sweet potatoes, sliced thin (the thinner the slice, the crisper the chip)

Cayenne pepper
   ***OR* paprika**
   ***OR* chili powder**

Preheat oven to 450°F.

Place sweet potato slices in single layer on nonstick cookie sheet (recipe will make two batches). For a touch of spice, sprinkle lightly with ONE of the suggested options. Bake 15 minutes, flipping once during baking. Remove from oven when chips are nicely browned. (The exact cooking time will depend on the thickness of the chips; keep an eye on them so they don't burn.) May be served hot or at room temperature.

Per Serving:
Calories: 125 **Fat:** 1g **Carbohydrate:** 27g **Protein:** 2g **Sodium:** 11mg

Embarrassingly Simple Rice

4 Servings

1 14-ounce can (approx.) fat-free, lower-sodium chicken broth
3/4 cup water
1/2 teaspoon dried thyme
1 medium onion, chopped
1 cup white rice

Put the broth and water in a medium saucepan and bring to a boil. Stir in thyme, onion, and rice, cover, and lower the heat. Cook over moderate heat until liquid is absorbed, about 25 minutes.

Per Serving:
Calories: 104   **Fat:** 0g   **Carbohydrate:** 23g
Protein: 3g   **Sodium:** 275mg

SODIUM ALERT!

If you are on a sodium-restricted diet, then use, for example, Health Valley "no salt added" chicken broth.

Interesting variation: Put 6 fresh mushrooms that have been washed and dried into the food processor. Process them so they are chopped very, very fine. Put them in a large, nonstick skillet. Add two tablespoons of water and cook over low heat, letting the juices escape. When the chopped mushrooms are dry, stir while they brown slightly. Add them to the broth and water (with the thyme and onions if you like), stir, then add the rice and cook as directed above. To be a little fancier, buy one of the wild rice/white rice blends that are on the market. Adjust amount of liquid according to the directions on the package. (This is a remarkable dish for company.)

Per Serving:
Calories: 104   **Fat:** 0g   **Carbohydrate:** 24g   **Protein:** 3g   **Sodium:** 276mg
(Same sodium alert!)

Orange Rice
4 Servings

You can cook rice in almost any liquid. Experiment for different flavors! Here we use orange juice, as well as pieces of orange, fruit being one of the no-fat flavor enhancers.

1 cup water
1 1/4 cups orange juice
1/4 cup chopped water chestnuts
1/2 orange, peeled and chopped
1 cup rice

Put water, juice, water chestnuts, and orange into a medium saucepan. Bring to boil, add rice, cover, and reduce heat. Cook over moderate heat until liquid is absorbed, about 25 minutes. Serve hot or at room temperature.

Per Serving:
Calories: 220   **Fat:** 0g   **Carbohydrate:** 50g   **Protein:** 3g   **Sodium:** 3mg

CHAPTER
13

Embarrassingly

Simple

Recipes

Green Orzo and Peas
6 Servings

"Looks like rice! Tastes like pasta! It's ORZO!"

1 14-ounce can (approx.) fat-free, lower-sodium chicken broth
1/4 cup water
1 medium onion, chopped
1/2 cup chopped fresh parsley
1 cup orzo (uncooked)
1 10-ounce package frozen peas, thawed

Bring broth and water to boil in medium saucepan. Add onion, parsley, and orzo. Reduce heat and simmer gently, uncovered, stirring occasion-ally. Continue cooking about 10 minutes, or until liquid is absorbed. Remove from heat and toss with peas, which will warm quickly from the pasta. Serve warm or at room tem-perature.

SODIUM ALERT!

If you are on a sodium-restricted diet, then use, for example, Health Valley "no salt added" chicken broth.

Per Serving:
Calories: 149   **Fat:** 0g   **Carbohydrate:** 28g
Protein: 7g   **Sodium:** 213mg

Jack Sprat's Rice with Black Beans
4 Servings

1 14-ounce can (approx.) fat-free, lower-sodium chicken broth
1/4 cup water
1/2 cup white wine
1 small onion, chopped
1 medium carrot, scraped and chopped
3/4 cup uncooked rice
1/2 16-ounce can black beans, rinsed and drained

Put broth, water, wine, onion, and carrot in a medium saucepan and bring to a boil. Add rice and beans, cover, and reduce heat. Cook until liquid is absorbed, about 30 minutes. (This can also be done in the oven, which is handy if your oven is the kind that will turn itself on before you get home. Just put everything in a 2-quart baking dish and set the timer so the rice and beans will bake for one hour at 350°F.)

> **SODIUM ALERT!**
>
> If you are on a sodium-restricted diet, then use, for example, Health Valley "no salt added" chicken broth, and Eden "very low sodium" canned beans.

Per Serving:
Calories: 177 **Fat:** 1g **Carbohydrate:** 37g
Protein: 5g **Sodium:** 390mg

Don't waste that other half can of beans!
Marinate remaining half can of beans in 2 tablespoons fat-free salad dressing. Store, covered, in the refrigerator. Throw beans on your salad the next day.

Embarrassingly

Simple

Recipes

Meat-Free Chili
4 Servings

*This is hot, hot, hot! If that's too hot, use regular canned tomatoes
instead and add cumin and chili powder to taste.*

2 15-ounce cans Tex-Mex Style Diced Stewed Tomatoes
1/2 15-ounce can pink beans, rinsed and drained
2 carrots, peeled and sliced
Chopped onion (optional)
Grated fat-free cheese (optional)

Put tomatoes, beans, and carrots in medium
saucepan. Simmer 20 minutes. Garnish with
onion and cheese if desired.

Per Serving:
Calories: 97   **Fat:** 2g   **Carbohydrate:** 18g
Protein: 4g   **Sodium:** 476mg

SODIUM ALERT!
If you are on a sodium restricted diet, then use, for example, Eden "no salt added" crushed tomatoes and Eden "very low sodium" canned beans. Add cumin and chili powder to taste.

Don't waste that other half can of beans!
Mash remaining half can of beans with a fork. Add hot sauce to taste.
Use as a dip. Serve with fat-free corn chips.

Chickpeas (Garbanzo Beans), Fast and Furious
4 Servings

Even if the idea of eating beans has never appealed to you, you might try this recipe. In just a couple of minutes you'll have a delicious side dish.

2 teaspoons olive oil

1 medium onion, chopped

2 cloves garlic, chopped fine, or 1 teaspoon of the garlic that comes in a cute little jar, all ready to use

1 16-ounce can chickpeas, rinsed and drained

Freshly ground pepper to taste

Heat the olive oil in a medium, nonstick skillet over moderate heat. Add the onion and garlic and sauté until translucent. Add chickpeas, toss quickly to heat through, and finish off with a dose of freshly ground pepper.

> **SODIUM ALERT!**
>
> If you are on a sodium-restricted diet, then use, for example, Eden "very low sodium" canned beans.

Per Serving:

Calories: 136 **Fat:** 4g **Carbohydrate:** 19g **Protein:** 6g   **Sodium:** 180mg

Embarrassingly

Simple

Recipes

Vegetables

W hen you are dealing with embarrassingly simple recipes, you can get a lot of mileage by using a variety of serving styles. We are referring to sleight-of-hand (not topless serving). You make a vegetable recipe one night, then the next night you make it slightly differently, change a little something, or maybe just serve on a different platter, and there you are with another dish altogether. Or you can use vegetables as a "bed" for a piece of chicken or fish; simply by changing the vegetables, you change the entire dish.

You can make VEGETABLES EVERY WAY with these seven simple methods. We've given examples of each.

1) *Roasting – modest (covered)*	Roasted Asparagus Golden Oldies
2) *Roasting – immodest (uncovered)*	Garlic-Roasted Carrots
3) *Sautéing – in a bit of broth*	Vegetable Combo
4) *Simmering – in a bath of broth*	Savoy Cabbage with Carrots Broccoli and Cauliflower
5) *Bubbling – in tomatoes*	Green Beans with Tomatoes
6) *Steaming – in a foil pouch*	Mushrooms in Foil
7) *Grilling – outdoors*	Grilled Zucchini

Roasted Asparagus

4 Servings

> **20 or 24 asparagus spears, depending on size**
> **2 teaspoons olive oil**
> **Freshly ground pepper to taste**
> **3 tablespoons minced fresh parsley**
> **Aluminum foil**

Preheat oven to 400°F.

Arrange asparagus in single layer on nonstick baking sheet. Drizzle with olive oil and season with pepper. Sprinkle with parsley, cover lightly with foil, and roast 15 minutes.

Per Serving:
Calories: 60   **Fat:** 3g   **Carbohydrate:** 10g   **Protein:** 0g   **Sodium:** 0mg

◆   ◆   ◆   ◆

Grilled Zucchini

4 Servings

Select tender, young zucchini, not the great big ones that could double as jugglers' clubs.

> **4 small-to-medium zucchini**
> **Nonstick cooking spray**
> **Dried herb seasoning**

Cut zucchini in half lengthwise. Spray cut side LIGHTLY, then sprinkle with herb seasoning. Lay cut side down on grill and cook about 15-20 minutes or until tender, turning once.

Per Serving:
Calories: 24   **Fat:** 0g   **Carbohydrate:** 5g   **Protein:** 1g   **Sodium:** 0mg

Embarrassingly

Simple

Recipes

Vegetable Combo

6 Servings

It's possible to brown foods without fat, and this recipe shows you how. Try other vegetables – bell peppers, for instance – the next time you make this.

1/4 cup canned vegetable broth
1 medium white onion (sweet), sliced
1 medium zucchini, cubed
1 medium yellow (summer) squash, cubed
6 fairly large fresh mushrooms, sliced
1 teaspoon fines herbes, dried
4 fresh medium plum tomatoes, cut up
Freshly ground pepper to taste

Put broth and onion in a large, nonstick skillet and simmer until onion is transparent. Add squash and mushrooms. Sprinkle with fines herbes. Let cook until liquid evaporates and vegetables start to brown a bit, about 10 to 15 minutes. Keep heat high and DON'T LEAVE THE PREMISES! Stir from time to time. Add tomatoes and stir as they cook into the vegetable mixture. Season with fresh pepper.

Per Serving:
Calories: 28 **Fat:** 0g **Carbohydrate:** 5g **Protein:** 2g **Sodium:** 77mg

Vegetable Bouquet

4 Servings

This has a lot in common with Vegetable Combo (page 158), but because this is roasted, there is no constant stirring required here.

4 medium red potatoes, cubed (not peeled)

1 red bell pepper, cubed, seeds removed

1 yellow bell pepper, cubed, seeds removed

1/2 pound medium mushrooms, quartered

4 cloves garlic, crushed, or 2 teaspoons of the garlic that comes in a cute little jar, all ready to use

2 teaspoons olive oil

2 teaspoons dried rosemary

Freshly ground pepper to taste

1 tablespoon balsamic vinegar

Cook potatoes in boiling water to cover for 10 minutes; drain. In large bowl, toss potatoes, peppers, and mushrooms, with garlic, olive oil, and rosemary. Spread in baking dish (lined with foil for easy cleanup). Season with pepper. Broil 2 inches from heat for 15 minutes until nicely browned, stirring every once in a while so vegetables brown evenly. Return to bowl and toss with vinegar. Serve hot or at room temperature.

Per Serving:

Calories: 267   **Fat:** 3g   **Carbohydrate:** 70g   **Protein:** 5g   **Sodium:** 0mg

Holiday Squash
4 Servings

1 acorn squash
Nonstick cooking spray
1 cup canned whole cranberry sauce

Preheat oven to 350°F.

Rinse squash and cut in quarters but do not peel. Scoop out seeds and pulp. (If this reminds you of your pumpkin-carving days, that's no accident, since acorn squash and pumpkins are in the same family.) Slice the four quarters, which will make little smile-shaped pieces. Spray baking dish LIGHTLY with cooking spray and lay squash pieces in dish. Spread with cranberry sauce. Bake uncovered for 45 minutes.

Per Serving:
Calories: 127   **Fat:** 0g   **Carbohydrate:** 30g   **Protein:** 2g   **Sodium:** 0mg

◆   ◆   ◆   ◆

Peas with a Twist
4 Servings

1 teaspoon olive oil
1 medium onion, chopped
1/2 teaspoon dried thyme
1 cup lettuce leaves, broken into small
    pieces (a variety of lettuces is nice)
1 1-pound can baby peas
Freshly ground pepper to taste

> **SODIUM ALERT!**
> If you are on a sodium-restricted diet, substitute frozen peas for canned. Cook according to package directions before proceeding with recipe.

Heat oil in nonstick pan. Add onion and cook until tender. Sprinkle with thyme, toss together, and add lettuce. Cook a minute or two, until lettuce wilts. Add peas, toss to heat through. Season with pepper.

Per Serving:
Calories: 79   **Fat:** 1g   **Carbohydrate:** 13g   **Protein:** 4g   **Sodium:** 200mg

Green Beans with Tomatoes

4 Servings

1 9-ounce package frozen cut green beans
1 14 ½-ounce can "recipe ready" diced tomatoes
1 6 ½-ounce can sliced mushrooms
Freshly ground pepper to taste

Preheat oven to 350°F.

Knock box of frozen beans against the counter to separate beans. Dump into 1-quart casserole dish with lid (foil will do if you have no lid). Open mushrooms, drain off juice, and add mushrooms to beans. Add tomatoes. Season with pepper. Cover with lid or foil and bake until beans are tender and dish is piping hot, 50-60 minutes.

Per Serving:
Calories: 62   **Fat:** 0g   **Carbohydrate:** 13g
Protein: 3g   **Sodium:** 436mg

CHAPTER
13

Embarrassingly

Simple

Recipes

> **SODIUM ALERT!**
>
> If you are on a sodium-restricted diet, substitute 2 cups chopped fresh tomatoes and 1 cup sliced fresh mushrooms. Steam mushrooms briefly before using in recipe.

Good Old Beans

4 Servings

*Unlike the previous recipe, this is a casserole-free way to fix green beans.
And we've chosen French cut beans this time.*

1 teaspoon olive oil

1 medium onion, chopped

**1 clove garlic, minced, or 1/2 teaspoon of the garlic that comes
in a cute little jar, all ready to use**

1 9-ounce package frozen French cut green beans, thawed

1 6 1/2-ounce can sliced mushrooms

Freshly ground pepper to taste

2 teaspoons lemon juice

Heat oil in medium nonstick skillet. Add onion and garlic, sauté until
tender, then add beans. Cook, stirring, over medium heat until just tender, about 6 or 7 minutes. Add mushrooms, juice and all. Stir another
minute or two, until mixture is heated through.
Transfer to bowl, season with pepper, then toss
with lemon juice. Serve hot or at room temperature.

Per Serving:

Calories: 49   **Fat:** 1g   **Carbohydrate:** 8g
Protein: 2g   **Sodium:** 200mg

> **SODIUM ALERT!**
>
> If you are on a
> sodium restricted
> diet, substitute 1
> cup sliced fresh
> mushrooms.
> Steam briefly
> before using in
> recipe.

Golden Oldies

4 Servings

Carrots and sweet potatoes have been around for a long time, but here they appear together, a new and delicious combination. The deep golden yellow makes them beautiful as well as tasty.

> **2 medium onions, chopped**
> **1 teaspoon olive oil**
> **1 cup baby carrots**
> **2 medium sweet potatoes, skinned and cubed**
> **1/2 cup water**
> **1 tablespoon brown sugar**

Preheat oven to 400°F.

Using a 1-quart casserole dish that is safe for use on the top of the stove, sauté the onion in the olive oil until transparent. Add carrots and potatoes, add water, and sprinkle with brown sugar. Cover with the casserole lid if there is one, or with foil if there isn't. Bake for 30 minutes, until vegetables are tender.

Per Serving:

Calories: 99   **Fat:** 1g   **Carbohydrate:** 21g   **Protein:** 1g   **Sodium:** 0mg

Embarrassingly

Simple

Recipes

Garlic-Roasted Carrots
4 Servings

1 ½ pounds baby carrots

**2 cloves garlic, crushed, or 1 teaspoon of the garlic that comes
in a cute little jar, all ready to use**

Freshly ground pepper to taste

Nonstick cooking spray

Preheat oven to 425°F.

Put carrots in bowl, add garlic and pepper, and toss to coat. Lay in baking dish (lined with foil for easy cleanup) in single layer, spray LIGHTLY with cooking spray, and roast 30-40 minutes, turning once, until tender and brown. Serve hot or at room temperature.

Per Serving:

Calories: 54   **Fat:** 0g   **Carbohydrate:** 12g   **Protein:** 2g   **Sodium:** 0mg

Broccoli and Cauliflower

4 Servings

Not so fast! Even if you're sure you don't like these vegetables, you may very well like them in this particular incarnation. It's a handy dish because you cook it in the oven, which leaves both hands free.

1 medium onion, sliced
4 stalks celery, sliced
3 cups combined "flowers" (the little flower tops, not the stems)
1 cup fat-free, lower-sodium chicken broth

Preheat oven to 400°F.

Spread onion and celery in medium casserole dish. Put "flowers" on top. Pour chicken broth over all, cover with lid or foil, and bake for 45 minutes.

Per Serving:
Calories: 44   **Fat:** 0g   **Carbohydrate:** 10g
Protein: 1g   **Sodium:** 320mg

SODIUM ALERT!

If you are on a sodium-restricted diet, then use, for example, Health Valley "no salt added" chicken broth.

Embarrassingly

Simple

Recipes

Fresh Spinach and Portobello Mushrooms
4 Servings

If you're lucky, you'll find the spinach in a cellophane bag that has been pre-washed. If so, add 1/4 cup of water to the skillet when you add the spinach. If you have to wash the spinach, enough water will cling to the leaves to make the extra water unnecessary.

> **1 teaspoon olive oil**
> **2 large cloves garlic, chopped, or 1 teaspoon of the garlic that comes in a cute little jar, all ready to use**
> **1 medium onion, chopped**
> **6 ounces fresh Portobello mushrooms, sliced**
> **1 10-ounce package fresh spinach, washed**
> **Freshly ground pepper to taste**

Heat olive oil in a large, nonstick skillet. Add garlic and onion; cook until translucent. Add mushroom slices and cook over medium heat until very soft, about 10 minutes. Add spinach (as well as extra water, if necessary). Cover with lid or foil. Allow to steam for another 10 minutes or so, until spinach is wilted but still bright green. Season with pepper and stir well.

Per Serving:
Calories: 50 **Fat:** 2g **Carbohydrate:** 5g **Protein:** 3g **Sodium:** 64mg

Spinach with Pizazz

6 Servings

"But I don't see any 'pizazz' in the list of ingredients!" we hear you say. Ah, but trust us. There's plenty in this dish, we promise.

> **2 10-ounce boxes frozen whole leaf spinach**
> **1 medium onion, chopped**
> **2 teaspoons cider vinegar**
> **1/2 cup fat-free sour cream**
> **Freshly ground pepper to taste**

Put spinach and onion in medium saucepan and cook according to directions on box. Drain well and return to pan. Add vinegar, sour cream, and pepper. Reheat briefly.

Per Serving:

Calories: 47   **Fat:** 0g   **Carbohydrate:** 2g   **Protein:** 3g   **Sodium:** 108mg

Embarrassingly

Simple

Recipes

Collard Greens on Air
4 Servings

This recipe opens up all sorts of "on Air" possibilities. Try, for instance, "Broccoli on Air." The chopped, frozen versions of collard greens and broccoli look remarkably alike, but collard greens have a stronger flavor than broccoli and are much chewier. Because of their enormous health benefits, they are definitely worth tasting if you've never tried them before.

12 fat-free saltines
1 cup fat-free milk
1 medium onion, chopped
1 tablespoon Worcestershire sauce
1/2 cup egg substitute
1 10-ounce box frozen chopped collard greens, cooked according to package directions
Freshly ground pepper to taste
Nonstick cooking spray

Preheat oven to 350°F.

Break up saltines into a medium bowl. (Enjoy it—the crumbling is actually kind of fun.) Add milk and soak briefly until soft. Add other ingredients and pour into small casserole dish LIGHTLY sprayed with cooking spray. Bake uncovered for 45 minutes.

SODIUM ALERT!

If you are on a sodium-restricted diet, use 6 salt-free saltines and 6 fat-free saltines.

Per Serving:
Calories: 107   **Fat:** 0g   **Carbohydrate:** 15g   **Protein:** 9g   **Sodium:** 184g

Mushrooms in Foil

4 Servings

Incredibly easy, no cleanup, and perfect as a side dish or as a "sauce" for fish or chicken. There's no need to add any liquid, because, as you'll see, the mushrooms have lots of juice.

> **1 pound fresh mushrooms (mix varieties if desired)**
> **Freshly ground pepper to taste**
> **Dried herb of your choice, such as oregano (optional)**
> **Heavy aluminum foil**

Preheat oven to 400°F.

Slice mushrooms and lay on foil. Sprinkle with pepper (and herbs, if you've decided to use them). Seal foil and bake for 15 to 20 minutes.

Per Serving:
Calories: 36 **Fat:** 0g **Carbohydrate:** 5g **Protein:** 4g **Sodium:** 20mg

Savoy Cabbage with Carrots
4 Servings

Even if you aren't a big cabbage fan, give savoy cabbage a try. Its flavor is much more delicate than that of the original.

1 small head savoy cabbage

1 14-ounce can (approx.) fat-free, lower-sodium chicken broth

1/2 1-pound package small, peeled carrots (available in super-market produce section)

1 teaspoon caraway seeds (optional)

Cut cabbage in quarters; remove core and discard. Rinse cabbage and slice thin. Put cabbage in a medium saucepan with the broth and carrots. Bring to a boil and reduce heat. Simmer, covered, until vegetables are tender, about 30 minutes. Sprinkle with caraway seeds if you feel like it.

Per Serving:
Calories: 77 **Fat:** 1g **Carbohydrate:** 13g
Protein: 4g **Sodium:** 275mg

SODIUM ALERT!

If you are on a sodium-restricted diet, then use, for example, Health Valley "no salt added" chicken broth.

"Mexican" Eggplant
4 Servings

Again, a casserole, convenient in that it can be fixed ahead.

1 15-ounce can tomato sauce

1 small to medium eggplant, unpeeled and sliced on the diagonal, giving you bigger, easier-to-layer slices

1/2 pound fresh mushrooms, sliced

1 medium white sweet onion, sliced

1 16-ounce can of pink (or other) beans, rinsed, drained, and puréed with 1/2 can of water

1/2 teaspoon dried cumin, puréed with beans (optional)

2 tablespoons chopped fresh chives (optional)

Preheat oven to 350°F.

Spread a bit of the tomato sauce in the bottom of a shallow baking dish (13 1/2" x 8 3/4" x 1 3/4"), and then start layering. First, the slices of eggplant. Then scatter some mushrooms and onion slices around. Add more of the tomato sauce. Make another layer of eggplant, mushroom, and onion slices. Before adding more tomato sauce, spread the puréed beans (that have been combined with cumin, if desired) and then top with the sauce. Bake for one hour, or until bubbly. Sprinkle fresh chives on top if you are using them.

> **SODIUM ALERT!**
>
> If you are on a sodium-restricted diet, then use, for example, Hunt's "no salt added" tomato sauce and Eden "very low sodium" canned beans.

Per Serving:
Calories: 167   **Fat:** 1g   **Carbohydrate:** 30g
Protein: 9g   **Sodium:** 710mg

Embarrassingly

Simple

Recipes

Soups & Salads

Cold days
Hot days
Soup days
Salad days

On those days when you have no time to fix dinner, consider soups and salads. They might dress up a meal, or they might actually be a meal.

Sneaky Bean Soup
"Floating Casserole" I
4 Servings

This soup is just the thing to get non-bean-eaters to eat beans. The beans are puréed and blended into the soup, and no one knows they are there. (Here we suggest using low-sodium canned beans, so that the per-serving sodium level of the soup will not be unacceptably high.)

1 14-ounce package soup vegetables (celery, parsnip, turnip, carrot, parsley, dill, et cetera, conveniently packaged and waiting for you in the produce section of your supermarket)

2 14-ounce cans (approx.) fat-free, lower-sodium chicken broth

1/2 cup water

1 16-ounce can "very low sodium" navy beans, such as Eden, rinsed and drained

Rinse, peel (as necessary), and chop all vegetables. Place in a large saucepan. Add broth. Bring to a boil, then simmer, covered, until tender, about 30 minutes. Meanwhile, add the water to the beans and purée in a food processor. At the end of the 30 minutes, add to the soup for thickening and great taste. Simmer 15 minutes longer.

Per Serving:
Calories: 184 **Fat:** 0g **Carbohydrate:** 38g
Protein: 8g **Sodium:** 593mg

SODIUM ALERT!

If you are on a sodium-restricted diet, then use, for example, Health Valley "no salt added" chicken broth.

CHAPTER 13

Embarrassingly

Simple

Recipes

Bean and Pasta Soup
"Floating Casserole" II
8 servings

This recipe calls for frozen spinach, which means you don't have to take the time to pick off the tough stems and then get the sand out of the leaves, but if you'd rather use fresh, that's great.

> **3 14-ounce cans (approx.) fat-free, lower-sodium chicken broth. (Save cans for measuring water.)**
>
> **3 cans water**
>
> **1/2 16-ounce box "ditalini" pasta (tiny pasta tubes)**
>
> **1 16-ounce can white kidney beans, rinsed and drained**
>
> **1 box frozen leaf spinach, thawed and drained (to thaw, put in colander and run under cold water)**

Put broth and water in a large saucepan. Bring to a boil, add pasta, reduce heat and cover. Cook until tender, about ten minutes. Add beans and spinach. Heat through.

Per Serving:
Calories: 157 **Fat:** 1g **Carbohydrate:** 30g
Protein: 7g   **Sodium:** 550mg

SODIUM ALERT!

If you are on a sodium-restricted diet, then use, for example, Health Valley "no salt added" chicken broth, and Eden "very low sodium" canned beans.

Split Pea Soup
"Floating Casserole" III
6 servings

This recipe uses dried split peas. Unlike most other dried beans, they do not need to be soaked in advance. They should, however, be checked for the presence of small pebbles.

This is a good, thick soup. It will thicken as it cools, giving it a kind of magical quality. Since you'll have to add water each time you heat the soup, it will replenish itself.

> **1 16-ounce package dried split peas**
> **2 ½ quarts water**
> **2 carrots, peeled and sliced, about 1 cup**
> **1 large onion, coarsely chopped**
> **1 large stalk celery, coarsely chopped, about 1/2 cup**
> **1 teaspoon salt**
> **1/2 teaspoon dried oregano**

Put everything in a large pot. Bring to a boil, then cover and simmer gently until thick, about 1 1/2 hours.

SODIUM ALERT!

If you are on a sodium-restricted diet, use your favorite salt substitute.

Per Serving:
Calories: 160   **Fat:** 0g **Carbohydrate:** 30g
Protein: 10g   **Sodium:** 427mg

Strawberry and Spinach Salad
4 Servings

Fruit, a no-fat flavor enhancer, is a wonderful, healthy addition to salad, and you'll find you need less dressing when you use it. As you'll see here, strawberries work well. You might also try melon (particularly in summer, when melons are so good), and apples (good all year long).

Make dressing first, so the flavors have a chance to blend:

> **1/4 cup canola oil**
> **2 tablespoons cider vinegar**
> **1 teaspoon dried onions**
> **1 teaspoon sugar**

Put all ingredients in a small jar, shake well, and set aside. Do this as far ahead as is convenient, so the flavors have a chance to blend.

The salad:

> **1 pint fresh strawberries (stems removed), sliced**
> **1 6-ounce bag prewashed baby spinach, or 1 10-ounce bag fresh spinach, washed well and stems removed**

Lay spinach on pretty platter and mound berries in the middle, allowing green to show around the edges. Just before serving, give dressing a final shake and pour carefully over the salad.

Per Serving:
Calories: 191   **Fat:** 15g   **Carbohydrate:** 19g   **Protein:** 1g   **Sodium:** 0mg

Cucumber Salad

4 Servings

2 large cucumbers
1/2 teaspoon sugar
2 tablespoons red wine vinegar
1 scallion, chopped (including green)
1/2 cup plain fat-free yogurt

Peel and seed cucumbers. (If you've never seeded one: Cut it in half lengthwise, then hollow it out, like a little canoe, by scraping out the seeds with a spoon.) Cube the cucumbers. Mix with the sugar, vinegar, and scallion. Let sit a few minutes, but stir occasionally. Put yogurt into a bowl, pour juice off cucumbers and into yogurt, combine well, and add cucumbers. Toss together.

Per Serving:
Calories: 15   **Fat:** 0g   **Carbohydrate:** 5g   **Protein:** 1g   **Sodium:** 20mg

Embarrassingly

Simple

Recipes

Embarrassingly

Simple

Recipes

Assembled Salad
4 Servings

You can use leftover chicken or fish instead of the tuna, if you prefer. Serve some crusty bread with this and it makes a nice, light meal.

12 small red-skinned potatoes (do not peel)
Lettuce leaves
1 8-ounce can French cut green beans
1 8-ounce can sliced red beets
1 12-ounce can tuna packed in water
1/4 cup Our Favorite Oil and Vinegar Dressing, page 189
2 eggs, hard boiled

Boil potatoes until tender, about 20 minutes. Allow to cool. Meanwhile, make a bed of lettuce leaves on a platter. Open cans and drain them. Separate egg yolks from whites. Discard yolks and quarter whites. Cut potatoes in half and arrange along with beans and beets on the lettuce, leaving space for tuna in the center. Drizzle dressing over all. Flake tuna in middle of vegetables. Garnish with egg white quarters.

Per Serving:
Calories: 334 **Fat:** 13g **Carbohydrate:** 28g **Protein:** 28g **Sodium:** 455mg

Updated Pasta Salad
4 Servings

Happily, fat is not an issue with pasta. And, because all pastas are made from pretty much the same ingredients and differ only in their shape, you can easily vary the look of your pasta dishes.

This is a good summer dish, best served at room temperature, and can be made ahead. Water chestnuts provide a nice crunch, and they don't contain fat. The dressing called for is Wish-Bone Lite Classic Dijon Vinaigrette, a bottled dressing with half the fat of regular.

A few slices of leftover Grilled Turkey Breast (see recipe, page 199) are a nice addition to this salad.

> **8 ounces interestingly shaped pasta, such as rotini or cavatelli, cooked just until done and rinsed to remove starch**
>
> **8 cherry tomatoes, halved**
>
> **1/2 8-ounce can sliced water chestnuts, drained**
>
> **4 leaves fresh basil, chopped**
>
> **2 tablespoons chopped red onion**
>
> **2 leaves raw spinach, washed, stems removed, and cut up with scissors**
>
> **4 large black olives, sliced thin**
>
> **1/2 cup Wish-Bone Lite Classic Dijon Vinaigrette**

Place pasta, cherry tomatoes, water chestnuts, basil, red onion, spinach and olives in a large bowl. Toss with dressing.

If you are making this ahead, refrigerate. Allow to return to room temperature before serving.

Per Serving:
Calories: 279 **Fat:** 7g **Carbohydrate:** 47g
Protein: 7g **Sodium:** 393mg

SODIUM ALERT!

If you are on a sodium-restricted diet, use a low-sodium, fat-free dressing, and skip the olives.

Tongue-Twister Pasta Salad: Scallops and Shells
4 Servings

There are two kinds of scallops, large ones ("sea" scallops) and small ones ("bay" scallops). We find it easy to remember which is which because we know that the sea (that is, the ocean) is larger than the bay.

> **1 pound bay scallops**
> **2 tablespoons lemon juice**
> **1/2 cup dry white wine**
> **1/2 cup water**
> **Freshly ground pepper taste**
>
> **8 ounces shell pasta, cooked, rinsed, and drained**
> **3/8 cup Our Favorite Oil and Vinegar Dressing, page 189**
> **OR**
> **1/2 cup Fat-Free "Pesto," page 191**
> **Garnishes for color (optional):**
> **1 medium tomato, chopped**
> **1 scallion, chopped**

Using a medium skillet, combine scallops with lemon juice, wine, and water. Cook over high heat, tossing scallops in the liquid so they cook evenly. Continue cooking until they turn white, which will take just a few minutes. Season with pepper, combine with pasta, and toss with dressing or pesto. Garnish with tomato and scallion, if desired. Serve at room temperature.

Per Serving:
Calories: 426 **Fat:** 14g **Carbohydrate:** 40g **Protein:** 30g **Sodium:** 25mg

Crunchy Tuna Salad

(Or use canned red salmon to make Salmon Salad)

2 Servings

> **1 6 ½ -ounce can solid white tuna in water**
> **2 tablespoons canned water chestnuts**
> **1 small carrot, chopped, about 2 tablespoons**
> **2 teaspoons chopped red onion**
> **1 tablespoon chopped celery**
> **1/4 cup fat-free plain yogurt**
> **1 teaspoon Dijon mustard**

Drain tuna, empty into a bowl, and mash with fork. Add water chestnuts, carrot, red onion and celery. Mix together. Combine yogurt and mustard, then add to tuna salad.

Per Serving:
Calories: 134   **Fat:** 2g **Carbohydrate:** 5g
Protein: 24g **Sodium:** 389mg

SODIUM ALERT!
If you are on a sodium-restricted diet, use a tuna such as Bumble Bee Diet Low Salt Chunk White Tuna packed in water, or Chicken of the Sea Diet Chunk Light Tuna packed in water.

If made with salmon:

Per Serving:
Calories: 196   **Fat:** 7g   **Carbohydrate:** 9g
Protein: 24g   **Sodium:** 552mg

SODIUM ALERT!
If you are on a sodium-restricted diet, use a salmon such as Season Blueback or Pink Salmon, "no salt added," or Feather-weight Pink Sal-mon, "no salt added."

Embarrassingly

Simple

Recipes

Herbed Potato Salad

4 Servings

1 ½ pounds small red-skinned potatoes, cubed (do not peel)
1 teaspoon olive oil
1 medium onion, chopped
1 teaspoon dried thyme
1 teaspoon dried basil
1/2 teaspoon dried oregano

Simmer potatoes in water until tender, about 15 minutes. Drain. While they are cooking, sauté onion in oil until tender. Combine potatoes with onion and herbs. Serve warm or at room temperature.

Per Serving:
Calories: 130   **Fat:** 1g   **Carbohydrate:** 31g   **Protein:** 4g   **Sodium:** 0mg

Sunset Potato Salad
4 Servings

1 ½ pounds sweet potatoes, peeled and cubed

4 scallions, chopped

1/2 cup fat-free sour cream

3/8 cup Our Favorite Oil and Vinegar Dressing (see recipe, page 189)

Simmer sweet potatoes in water just until tender, about 10 minutes. Drain. Put in bowl with scallions. Combine sour cream and dressing. Toss with sweet potatoes.

Per Serving:

Calories: 275   **Fat:** 13g   **Carbohydrate:** 36g   **Protein:** 3g   **Sodium:** 40mg

Variation:

Skip the potatoes and substitute CAULIFLOWER. Steam the "flowers" from about half a head until tender, then continue as before.

Per Serving:

Calories: 182   **Fat:** 13g   **Carbohydrate:** 12g   **Protein:** 3g   **Sodium:** 40mg

Embarrassingly

Simple

Recipes

Rose-Rice Salad

4 Servings

1 cup water
1 1/4 cups low-sodium V-8 juice
1 medium onion, chopped
1/2 cup chopped water chestnuts
1 15-ounce can Veg-All
1 cup rice

Using medium saucepan, bring water, juice, onion, and water chestnuts to a boil. Stir in Veg-All and rice. Cover and reduce heat. Cook over medium heat until liquid is absorbed, about 25 minutes. Serve at room temperature.

Per Serving:

Calories: 235   **Fat:** 0g   **Carbohydrate:** 51g
Protein: 5g   **Sodium:** 304mg

SODIUM ALERT!

If you are on a sodium-restricted diet, use frozen mixed vegetables instead of Veg-All. Cook according to package directions before proceeding with recipe.

Marinated Beans and Vegetables

4 Servings

1 10-ounce box frozen mixed vegetables

1 16-ounce can chickpeas or other beans, rinsed and drained

2 tablespoons finely chopped red onion

1/4 cup Pritikin Fat-Free Dijon Balsamic or Fat-Free Honey French bottled dressing

Empty vegetables into a strainer and rinse with cold water. Put in a bowl with beans and onion. Pour dressing over all and mix well. Cover and allow to marinate for an hour or more on the counter, or overnight in the refrigerator.

SODIUM ALERT!

If you are on a sodium-restricted diet, then use, for example, Eden "very low sodium" canned beans.

Per Serving:

Calories: 193 **Fat:** 1g **Carbohydrate:** 37g
Protein: 9g **Sodium:** 260mg

CHAPTER 13

Embarrassingly

Simple

Recipes

Appetizers, Dressings, and Sauces

• • • •

Salmon Spread Appetizer

Makes about 1 cup

> 1 7 1/2-ounce can red salmon
> 1/2 teaspoon capers
> 1 tablespoon chopped water chestnuts
> 1 teaspoon chopped cocktail onions
> 1 tablespoon fat-free Thousand Island salad dressing

Drain salmon and remove any visible (dark) skin, as well as the small, round bone you'll probably find. Mash salmon with fork. Add dressing and mix well. Serve with fat-free crackers or chips.

Per Tablespoon:
Calories: 26   **Fat:** 1g   **Carbohydrate:** 1g   **Protein:** 3g   **Sodium:** 94mg

Eggplant and Tomato Spread

(puréed and delicious)

Makes about 2 cups

1 large eggplant

1 small onion, chopped fine

1 clove garlic, chopped fine, or 1/2 teaspoon of the garlic that comes in a cute little jar, all ready to use

1/4 cup chopped fresh parsley

1 large tomato, peeled and chopped (Dip tomato briefly in boiling water; it will peel easily.)

1 tablespoon lemon juice

Freshly ground pepper to taste

Preheat oven to 450°F.

Pierce eggplant with a fork and bake until very soft, about 1/2 hour. While eggplant is cooking, put onion, garlic, parsley, and tomato in a small, nonstick skillet lightly sprayed with oil. Cook slowly until vegetables are soft.

When eggplant is fully cooked, allow to cool before handling, unless you are blessed with asbestos hands. Then cut it in half lengthwise and scrape pulp out of shell into bowl of food processor. Add vegetables and purée the whole thing. Stir in lemon juice and pepper. Serve with fat-free crackers or chips.

Per Tablespoon:
Calories: 6 **Fat:** 0g **Carbohydrate:** 1g   **Protein:** 0g **Sodium:** 1mg

Embarrassingly

Simple

Recipes

Sun-dried Tomato Paste
Makes about 3/4 cup

Spread on fat-free crackers, this makes a delicious hors d'oeuvre. It's also great on chicken (see Chicken with Sun-Dried Tomato Paste, page 194).

1 8-ounce jar sun-dried tomatoes marinated in olive oil, very well drained
1 scallion, coarsely chopped
Freshly ground pepper

Put the sun-dried tomatoes and scallion in food processor bowl. Add a generous dose of pepper. Process until smooth.

Per Tablespoon:
Calories: 44 **Fat:** 3g **Carbohydrate:** 4g **Protein:** 1g **Sodium:** 6mg

A note on sun-dried tomatoes: Not only do they come marinated in oil, but also dried, in little cellophane packages. If you choose the dried ones (for salads and other dishes), don't try using them as is! They'll be harder to chew than tomato-flavored cardboard, and will taste like it, too. To soften: put tomatoes in a microwave container with enough water to cover them. Then "nuke" them, as the kids say, for 3 minutes. If you prefer (or have no microwave), put tomatoes in a small saucepan and cover with water. Bring to a boil, reduce heat, and simmer for about 5 minutes, or until tomatoes are very soft.

Our Favorite Oil and Vinegar Dressing
For 4 Servings of Salad (Makes 3/8 cup)

Embarrassingly

Simple

Recipes

A typical salad dressing can be a part of low-fat living. If you generally go with low-fat and fat-free foods, you can use a delicious, "regular-fat" dressing on your salad. There's method in our madness, because when you eat salad, you are eating vegetables. (Just remember that this is a salad dressing, not a salad dousing.)

  1/4 cup olive oil
  2 tablespoons balsamic or red wine vinegar
  1 teaspoon Dijon mustard
  Freshly ground pepper to taste

Combine all ingredients in a small jar. Shake well.

Per Serving:
Calories: 126 **Fat:** 14g **Carbohydrate:** 0g **Protein:** 0g **Sodium:** 17mg

Fat-free Gravy
Makes 2 Cups (8 Servings)

You don't have to give up gravy! Fat is a significant part of most gravy recipes, but not this one.

1 14-ounce can (approx.) fat-free, lower-sodium chicken broth
2 tablespoons cornstarch
1/4 cup water
1 teaspoon dried herbs, such as thyme or marjoram
Freshly ground pepper
1/4 teaspoon Kitchen Bouquet (for color)
Tabasco sauce (optional)

Bring the broth to a boil in a small saucepan. Meanwhile, stir the cornstarch into the water and mix well until dissolved. Using a wire whisk, add slowly to boiling broth, which will quickly thicken. Simmer a bit longer, just until gravy is clear and bubbly. Stir in herbs and pepper. Add Kitchen Bouquet. For gravy with a "bite," add a few drops of Tabasco to taste.

Per Serving:
Calories: 12   **Fat:** 0g **Carbohydrate:** 3g **Protein:** 0g   **Sodium:** 137mg

Yogurt-Mustard Sauce

Makes 1/2 cup

This "sauce" makes a good dip for fresh vegetables, a tasty salad dressing, a fine marinade, and a wonderful accompaniment for fish (poached salmon, for example), cold or hot.

> **1/2 cup fat-free plain yogurt**
> **1 teaspoon Dijon mustard**
> **1 ½ teaspoons fresh dill, chopped (Use only the thin, needle-like part, not the stems.)**

Blend and taste. If you prefer more or less mustard, adjust proportions accordingly.

Per Tablespoon:
Calories: 16 **Fat:** 0g **Carbohydrate:** 2g **Protein:** 2g **Sodium:** 39mg

◆   ◆   ◆   ◆

Fat-Free "Pesto"

Makes 1 cup (approximately 8 servings)

> **2 cups fresh basil leaves, stems removed (packed tightly)**
> **1/2 cup fat-free salad dressing (the vinaigrette type, NOT the creamy type)**
> **Freshly ground pepper to taste**

Put basil and salad dressing into food processor and process until smooth. Season with pepper.

Per Serving:
Calories: 12 **Fat:** 0g **Carbohydrate:** 2.5g **Protein:** .5g **Sodium:** 20mg

Embarrassingly

Simple

Recipes

Chicken & Turkey

Next come the EMBARRASSINGLY SIMPLE chicken and turkey recipes. Various things happen to the chicken. Each recipe serves four and therefore requires four small halves of boneless, skinless chicken breasts. These serving sizes are probably smaller than you are used to. When you are at the supermarket, standing in front of the poultry case, look for a package that contains 4 such breasts, for a total weight of 1 pound. When cooked, the breasts will weigh about 3 ounces each.

"Roadrunner"

4 Servings

Olive oil is the only added fat in this recipe. Crushed tomatoes and lemon juice, of course, contain no fat, and provide the flavorful liquid in which the chicken "steams."

4 small (4-ounce) halves chicken breast, boneless and skinless

Dried herb seasoning

1 small onion, chopped

1 clove garlic, minced fine, or 1/2 teaspoon of the garlic that comes in a cute little jar, all ready to use

2 teaspoons olive oil

1 teaspoon lemon juice

1 14-ounce can crushed tomatoes

Preheat oven to 350°F.

Rinse chicken under cold running water. Pat dry with paper towel and lay in baking dish in single layer. Season to taste with the dried herb seasoning.

Using a small, nonstick skillet, sauté onion and garlic in olive oil until translucent. Sprinkle on top of chicken. Add lemon juice to crushed tomatoes and pour over all. Cover with foil and bake for 45 minutes.

> **SODIUM ALERT!**
>
> If you are on a sodium-restricted diet, then use, for example, Eden "no salt added" crushed tomatoes.

Per Serving:

Calories: 193 **Fat:** 5g **Carbohydrate:** 8g **Protein:** 27g **Sodium:** 350mg

Embarrassingly

Simple

Recipes

Chicken with Sun-dried Tomato Paste
4 Servings

Cooking with wine is one of the fat-free cooking methods. And foil keeps the chicken juicy.

4 small (4-ounce) halves chicken breast, boneless and skinless

4 teaspoons sun-dried tomato paste (see recipe, page 188)

1/4 cup white wine

Heavy aluminum foil large enough to make envelope around chicken

Preheat oven to 350°F.

Rinse chicken breasts in cold water; pat dry with paper towel. Lay in single layer on foil. Spread sun-dried tomato paste on each piece, pour wine around chicken, seal foil, place in a baking dish, and bake for 45 minutes.

Per Serving:
Calories: 193   **Fat:** 5g   **Carbohydrate:** 8g   **Protein:** 27g   **Sodium:** 63mg

All-Purpose Chicken
4 Servings

This is a pleasantly moist, plain chicken that may be used "as is," and is also wonderful for all sorts of other things: chicken salad, sandwiches, and as a topping for a green salad.

You'll see that this recipe bears a startling resemblance to Chicken with Sun-dried Tomato Paste, but that's the way it is with these things. When you are cooking embarrassingly simple food, you find that minor recipe changes result in major taste differences.

4 small (4-ounce) halves chicken breast, boneless and skinless

Dried herb mixture (*OR* chili powder *OR* curry powder if you prefer)

Heavy aluminum foil large enough to make envelope around chicken

Preheat oven to 350°F.

Rinse chicken breasts in cold water; pat dry with paper towel. Lay in single layer on foil. Sprinkle with the dried herb mixture OR the chili powder OR the curry powder, seal foil, place in a baking dish and bake for 45 minutes.

Per Serving:
Calories: 135 **Fat:** 3g **Carbohydrate:** 0g **Protein:** 27g **Sodium:** 63mg

Embarrassingly

Simple

Recipes

Unlikely Chicken
4 Servings

This recipe combines three no-fat flavor enhancers: yogurt, fruit pre-serves, and mustard. Put them all together, and they look rather – ahem – strange. Just goes to show that you can't always judge a recipe by reading it! This is good hot or cold, and kids love it.

4 small (4-ounce) halves chicken breast, boneless and skinless
1/3 cup fat-free plain yogurt
1/3 cup apricot or raspberry all-fruit preserves
1 tablespoon Dijon mustard

Preheat oven to 350°F.

Rinse chicken breasts in cold water; pat dry with paper towel. Place in a small, shallow baking dish in a single layer. Combine yogurt, preserves, and mustard (we know, we know, but trust us), spread over the chicken breasts, and bake uncovered for 45 minutes.

Per Serving:
Calories: 219 **Fat:** 3g **Carbohydrate:** 21g **Protein:** 27g **Sodium:** 83mg

Chicken Marinated in Yogurt
4 Servings

Because you are using fat-free yogurt, there's no added fat in this recipe. Also you'll see that yogurt makes a great marinade and gives the cooked chicken a nice brown crust.

4 small (4-ounce) halves chicken breast, boneless and skinless

1/2 cup fat-free plain yogurt

1 clove garlic, chopped fine, or 1/2 teaspoon of the garlic that comes in a cute little jar, all ready to use

1 teaspoon dried mint

Freshly ground pepper to taste

Rinse chicken breasts in cold water; pat dry with paper towel. Combine yogurt, garlic, and mint in a bowl. Add chicken, tossing to coat well with yogurt. Add pepper and stir well. Refrigerate several hours or overnight, allowing to marinate. When dinnertime rolls around, as it has a way of doing, broil 7 minutes on each side.

Per Serving:
Calories: 151 **Fat:** 3g **Carbohydrate:** 2g **Protein:** 29g **Sodium:** 88mg

Embarrassingly

Simple

Recipes

Macaroni and...Chicken
4 Servings

Fooled you, didn't we? Well, you knew you wouldn't find a macaroni-and-cheese recipe in here! Like the casseroles of the 1950's, this uses up leftover chicken (or turkey), and if you have none left over, you can buy Perdue "Short Cuts," which amount to the same thing.

Preheat oven to 350°F.

1/2 16-ounce box elbow macaroni
3 tablespoons cornstarch
1 14-ounce can (approx.) fat-free, lower-sodium chicken broth
2 cups cut-up leftover chicken (or turkey)
1 10-ounce box frozen chopped broccoli, thawed
1/4 cup fat-free milk
1 tablespoon dried shallots (or onions)
Freshly ground pepper to taste

Cook macaroni just until tender. Drain, rinse, and transfer to casserole dish. Toss with chicken and broccoli. Next, put cornstarch into small saucepan, add 1/4 cup of the chicken broth, and stir until COMPLETELY BLENDED. Pour in rest of broth and heat, stirring, until sauce is thickened and smooth. Add milk, shallots, and pepper. Add sauce to macaroni, chicken, and broccoli, blend well, and cover casserole with lid or foil. Heat until piping hot, about 30 minutes. If you can't get everyone to the table just yet, reduce heat to 250°F until you can.

Per Serving:
Calories: 381 **Fat:** 4g **Carbohydrate:** 51g **Protein:** 33g **Sodium:** 277mg

Grilled Turkey Breast
4 Servings

The boneless, skinless turkey breast has come to the supermarket. It makes a nice change from the usual roasted affair, the recipe for which you can find in more than a few cookbooks. This recipe looks longer than the others but it's still very easy. Yogurt is used as a marinade, which moistens and flavors the turkey while you're off doing something else.

In order to make 4 servings, you need a 1-pound package of boneless turkey breast, but you will probably only find one that weighs a bit more, maybe "1.33 pounds" or so. This will give you leftovers to add to Updated Pasta Salad (see recipe, page 179).

1 1-pound package turkey breast (weight approximate), boneless and skinless

1 tablespoon lemon juice

MARINADE:

1 cup plain, fat-free yogurt

1 teaspoon celery seed

2 garlic cloves, crushed, or 1 teaspoon of the garlic that comes in a cute little jar, all ready to use

1/2 teaspoon freshly ground pepper

Other herbs and spices of your choice (optional)

When you get home and take the turkey breast out of the package, it won't look wildly appetizing, but don't despair. Rinse it in cold water, then pat dry with paper towel. Cut two little slashes in turkey and put it in a flat baking dish. Put a bit of the lemon juice in each slash. Some will spill over, but don't worry about that.

Combine marinade ingredients and coat the turkey. Cover and refrigerate, allowing to marinate for several hours or overnight, turning once. (No need to set your alarm to wake you in the middle of the night. Flip it when you get up for breakfast.) Then cook on a grill (with a hood), for 30 minutes, turning once. Keep hood closed while turkey is cooking. If your grill has a heat adjustment, use "medium." If not, set the rack a bit away from the coals.

If you don't have access to a grill, you can broil the turkey breast instead, probably about 20 minutes on each side, but the time will depend on thickness. The breast is done when you poke a fork into it and the juices run clear, not pink.

When the turkey is completely cooked, allow to cool for a few minutes to make slicing easier. Also good served at room temperature.

Per Serving:
Calories: 183 **Fat:** 3g **Carbohydrate:** 5g **Protein:** 34g **Sodium:** 104mg

Turkey Burger of Summer

4 Servings

Make sure the package says "Ground Turkey Breast," so you'll know you're getting the least amount of fat possible.

Dehydrated soup greens are rather expensive, so you might look for the cheaper "dried vegetable flakes," which are not, unfortunately, sold in supermarkets or grocery stores. Sometimes you'll see them in discount stores. You used to see them in the 5 and 10, but we all know what happened to the 5 and 10.

>   1 pound ground turkey breast
>   1 small onion, chopped
>   1/4 cup egg substitute
>   1/4 teaspoon garlic powder
>   1 tablespoon dried soup greens (found with the seasonings in the grocery store)
>   Freshly ground pepper to taste

You'll have to bring those soup greens back to life before you can use them. Put one tablespoon into a cup, add 3 tablespoons of water, then stick it in the microwave for 2-3 minutes, depending on your microwave.

Meanwhile, unwrap the ground turkey breast and dump it into a large bowl. Add the onion, egg substitute, garlic powder, and fresh pepper. Blend with fork. When the soup greens have revived, add them to the mixture and blend together. Shape into 4 patties. Put on the grill and cook, turning once after 7 minutes. Cook for a total of about 15 minutes, or until burgers are cooked through. Serve with mustard, ketchup, onion, whatever you like.

Per Serving:
Calories: 182 **Fat:** 4g **Carbohydrate:** 2g **Protein:** 33g **Sodium:** 32mg

Fish

Fish is wonderful for a low-fat diet and offers welcome variety. *Note that timing is important when cooking fish, and that cooking any fish too long results in something that is dry, firm, tasteless, and generally just plain unappealing.*

◆　◆　◆　◆

Carefree Flounder
4 Servings

This recipe uses three no-fat flavor enhancers: mustard, lemon (fruit) juice, and wine. The most time-consuming part of the recipe is unwrapping the fish.

> **1 pound fresh flounder fillets**
> **4 teaspoons Dijon mustard**
> **2 tablespoons lemon juice**
> **1/3 cup white wine**

Preheat oven to 350°F.

Lay the flounder in a single layer in a baking dish. Spread with mustard. Pour lemon juice and wine over all, and bake for 20 minutes. (If this strikes you as being just a little too simple, cut up a carrot, a medium tomato, and half a small onion. Put on top of fish before you put it in the oven.)

Per Serving:
Calories: 124　**Fat:** 1g　**Carbohydrate:** 1g　**Protein:** 17g　**Sodium:** 126mg

Salmon Cooked in Foil

4 Servings

Cooking in foil holds in juices and has the added advantage of leaving you with a pan that needs little or no scrubbing.

1 pound fresh salmon fillet (ask to have any large bones removed)

1 scallion, chopped

4 pieces sun-dried tomatoes that come marinated in olive oil; drained well and blotted with paper towels, then snipped in strips

1 tablespoon fresh tarragon (or other herb of your choice), snipped in small pieces

1/4 cup dry white wine

Freshly ground pepper to taste

Heavy aluminum foil, large enough to make an envelope around fish

Preheat oven to 450°F.

Lay salmon on foil. Sprinkle with scallion, sun-dried tomatoes, and tarragon (or other herb). Grind fresh pepper over all. Carefully pour wine over fish, seal aluminum pouch, lay in ovenproof dish and bake for 25 minutes.

Per Serving:
Calories: 198 **Fat:** 7g **Carbohydrate:** 3g **Protein:** 22g **Sodium:** 85mg

VARIATION: Lay the salmon on foil, sprinkle with 1 tablespoon fines herbes, dried, and freshly ground pepper. Seal foil and cook as above. (This is so good cold that you might want to just prepare it ahead and refrigerate, foil and all, for later use. Delicious served with Yogurt-Mustard Sauce, see recipe, page 191).

Per Serving:
Calories: 151 **Fat:** 7g **Carbohydrate:** 0g **Protein:** 22g **Sodium:** 48mg

Embarrassingly

Simple

Recipes

Grilled Salmon

4 Servings

1 tablespoon plus 1 teaspoon honey
1 teaspoon Dijon mustard
1 pound fresh salmon fillet

Combine honey and mustard. Lay salmon skin-side down on plate and spread honey-mustard mixture on top. Place on grill, skin-side down again, over medium flame. Cook 15 minutes, turn and cook another few minutes, just enough to brown other side. This side will burn easily because of the sauce, so be careful!

Per Serving:
Calories: 185   **Fat:** 9g   **Carbohydrate:** 1g   **Protein:** 23g   **Sodium:** 0mg

◆   ◆   ◆   ◆

Baked Mackerel

4 Servings

Marinating for even a short time makes the fish especially moist and flavorful.

1 pound fresh mackerel fillets
2 tablespoons lemon juice
1/2 teaspoon dried rosemary
1/2 teaspoon dried thyme
Freshly ground pepper to taste

Place fish in single layer, skin side down, in a shallow baking dish. Drizzle lemon juice over fish; sprinkle with herbs and fresh pepper. Cover dish with foil and refrigerate for an hour or more. About 30 minutes before you plan to start cooking, set the dish on the counter.

Preheat oven to 450°F. Bake for 20 minutes.

Per Serving:
Calories: 125   **Fat:** 5g   **Carbohydrate:** 0g   **Protein:** 20g   **Sodium:** 56mg

Monkfish, "The Poor Man's Lobster"
4 Servings

Embarrassingly

Simple

Recipes

Monkfish is known as "the poor man's lobster" because it's a whole lot cheaper but has a similar texture. Monkfish, however, has earned a good reputation all on its own, as this recipe demonstrates. Tomato and wine are the no-fat flavor enhancers.

> **1 pound monkfish fillets**
> **Nonstick cooking spray**
> **1 medium onion, chopped**
> **2 garlic cloves, crushed, or 1 teaspoon of the garlic that comes in a cute little jar, all ready to use**
> **1 medium tomato, chopped**
> **1/4 cup dry white wine**
> **Freshly ground pepper to taste**

Slice monkfish into 1-inch pieces. Spray a medium nonstick skillet LIGHTLY with cooking spray. Over medium high heat, sauté onion and garlic until lightly browned. Add fish and brown on both sides, which will only take a couple of minutes. Reduce heat slightly and add chopped tomato. Magically a sauce will begin to form (okay, it's really the juice from the monkfish); add the wine. Simmer everything for another 10-15 minutes, until fish is cooked through.

Per Serving:
Calories: 144 **Fat:** 2g **Carbohydrate:** 2g **Protein:** 25g **Sodium:** 0mg

Embarrassingly

Simple

Recipes

Zesty Halibut
4 Servings

Halibut is a pleasant white fish with something of a bland personality. It enjoys the company of strong flavors. Lemon, tomato, and wine are the no-fat flavor enhancers.

Nonstick cooking spray
1 medium onion, sliced thin
1 pound halibut fillet
1/2 lemon, sliced thin
1 medium tomato, chopped
1/2 cup dry white wine

Spray a medium baking dish LIGHTLY with cooking spray. Lay onion slices in bottom and the fish on top. Place lemon slices on fish and sprinkle with tomato. Season with pepper. Pour wine over all. Slowly bring to a boil on top of the stove, then transfer to oven and cook 10-15 minutes, until fish is cooked through.

Per Serving:
Calories: 153   **Fat:** 2g   **Carbohydrate:** 2g   **Protein:** 25g   **Sodium:** 0mg

Shrimp with Tomatoes
4 Servings

You'll want to use fresh, not frozen, shrimp for this.   Shrimp is very low in fat and, in moderate amounts, good for a heart-healthy diet. Serving the shrimp and tomatoes over rice helps to keep the amount moderate. While you're at it, why not try brown rice, which has the well-earned reputation of being particularly good for you? If you think of brown rice as being sticky and chewy, try Uncle Ben's Original Brown rice. It is neither of the above, and it tastes very good.

> **1/4 cup lemon juice**
>
> **2 teaspoons olive oil**
>
> **2 cloves garlic, crushed, or 1 teaspoon of the garlic that comes in a cute little jar, all ready to use**
>
> **1 pound medium fresh shrimp, peeled (about 32 shrimp)**
>
> **1 28-ounce can crushed tomatoes**
>
> **Freshly ground pepper to taste**

Combine lemon juice, olive oil, and garlic in a small bowl. Toss with shrimp. Cover with plastic wrap. Allow to marinate several hours in the refrigerator. (If you decide late in the day to make this, set bowl on counter for 1/2 hour before cooking.)

Remove shrimp from marinade and add liquid to tomatoes. Heat tomato mixture in a medium saucepan. While it is heating, cook shrimp by stir-frying them in a well-heated nonstick skillet for about 3 minutes or so. Allow to brown slightly. Add to tomatoes and season with pepper. Serve over rice.

SODIUM ALERT!

If you are on a sodium-restricted diet, then use, for example, Eden "no salt added" crushed tomatoes.

Per Serving (without rice):
Calories: 147   **Fat:** 3g **Carbohydrate:** 10g
Protein: 20g   **Sodium:** 570mg

Embarrassingly

Simple

Recipes

Desserts

I f the word "dessert" brings to mind "creamy," "rich," and "gooey," and only words like "lemonade" bring to mind "light" and "refreshing," you might want to re-think things. Desserts, too, can be light and refreshing. In fact, that's the trend. Times are changing, and this is a good time to consider changing along with them. There are many wonderful desserts in this section that are light and refreshing — and delicious.

What follows are desserts real people can eat every day. Many are made with fruit, and, if you find yourself getting rounder and rounder, this is clearly the way to go at dessert time. It's also a great way to get extra fruit into your day.

Also, there are fruit desserts here that are not only tasty but also beautiful and elegant enough for the fanciest party. Oh - did we mention they are embarrassingly simple? What else would you expect?

Embarrassingly

Simple

Recipes

Peaches in Wine

4 Servings

When served in a beautiful, stemmed glass, this makes a truly elegant dessert. Of course, it's equally delicious in a plastic cup. In any event, this is not a bad way to eat fruit!

2 16-ounce cans "lite" sliced peaches
1/2 cup dry red wine
4 Amaretti cookies (crunchy almond cookies), crushed for garnish

Drain peaches and put into bowl. Add wine. Allow to sit, stirring from time to time. Divide peaches among four pretty dessert glasses, adding a bit of wine to each glass. Top with crushed Amaretti cookies.

Per Serving:
Calories: 100 **Fat:** 0g **Carbohydrate:** 22g **Protein:** 0g **Sodium:** 8mg

Bizarre Strawberries

6 Servings

The small amount of balsamic vinegar is enough to bring out the flavor of the berries, making them surprisingly tasty.

(Note: You can cut the recipe in half and use Bizarre Strawberries to "garnish" another dessert—like "New Fashioned" Bread Pudding, for instance.)

> **1 quart fresh strawberries, stems removed**
> **4 teaspoons balsamic vinegar (a good, aged one)**

Rinse berries. Slice and put in attractive bowl. Sprinkle with vinegar.

Per Serving:
Calories: 37   **Fat:** 0g   **Carbohydrate:** 8g   **Protein:** 1g   **Sodium:** 0mg

◆   ◆   ◆   ◆

Bizarre Strawberries II

6 Servings

> **1 quart fresh strawberries, stems removed**
> **2 tablespoons lemon juice**
> **1/4 cup plus 2 tablespoons dry white wine**
> **1/4 cup powdered sugar**

Rinse berries. Slice and put in small bowl. In another bowl, mix lemon juice, wine, and sugar; stir until sugar dissolves completely. Pour over berries. Toss from time to time so that all the berries can absorb all the flavors.

Per Serving:
Calories: 74   **Fat:** 0g   **Carbohydrate:** 14g   **Protein:** 1g   **Sodium:** 0mg

Embarrassingly

Simple

Recipes

Bizarre Strawberries III

6 Servings

When you find yourself in an incredible hurry but simply have to produce a decent dessert, this first cousin of Bizarre Strawberries II is absolutely wonderful. It looks beautiful, too. Things don't come any easier than this.

1 quart fresh strawberries, stems left on
Small bowl of dry white wine
Small bowl of powdered sugar

Rinse berries and put in a pretty bowl. Set bowls of wine and powdered sugar alongside. Berries should be dipped first in wine, then in sugar.

Per Serving:
Calories: 74   **Fat:** 0g   **Carbohydrate:** 14g   **Protein:** 1g   **Sodium:** 0mg

Sweet Fruit Dessert

4 Servings

If you are using grapes for this, you can use either red or green seedless ones. In fact, a mixture looks very nice.

> **2/3 cup fat-free sour cream**
> **1/4 cup brown sugar**
> **3 cups seedless grapes or blueberries**

Mix sour cream and brown sugar until very well blended. Toss with fruit.

Per Serving:

Calories: 111   **Fat:** 0g   **Carbohydrate:** 25g   **Protein:** 2g   **Sodium:** 0mg

Embarrassingly

Simple

Recipes

Pretty Apple Dessert with Three Options
4 Servings

This is a "three in one" recipe. For company, offer all three versions.

4 large hard, crunchy apples (Winesap, for example)
1/4 cup all-fruit apricot preserves
OR   **1/4 teaspoon ground cinnamon mixed with 1 1/2 teaspoons sugar**
OR   **1/2 cup A Great Raspberry Sauce** (see recipe, page 220)

Peel and slice apples. Arrange in single layer on nonstick baking sheet. Broil (not too near heat) until golden, about 15 minutes. If you will be using the preserves, melt over low heat while apples are cooking.

Arrange browned apple slices in a pie pan. Pour preserves over them OR sprinkle with the cinnamon-sugar mixture OR top with raspberry sauce. Serve warm.

Per Serving:
Calories: 128 **Fat:** 0g **Carbohydrate:** 32g **Protein:** 0g   **Sodium:** 9mg

"FIRE AND ICE" Burnished Banana

1 Serving

This is the essence of "embarrassingly simple." It's even simple to increase the recipe according to how many people you are serving.

1 banana (not quite ripe? No problem)
1/2 to 1 teaspoon honey, depending on desired sweetness
1/2 teaspoon dark rum (optional)
Spoon

Preheat oven to 400°F.

Lay UNPEELED banana directly on oven rack and roast for 15 minutes. The skin will turn a beautiful, uniform black-brown, and the inside will be soft. Using a sharp paring knife, slit from one end to the other and drizzle in the honey, plus the rum if desired. Eat with the spoon.

Per Serving:
Calories: 121 **Fat:** 0g **Carbohydrate:** 30g **Protein:** 1.3g **Sodium:** 0mg

◆ ◆ ◆ ◆

"FIRE AND ICE" Frozen Banana

1 Serving

This is a good recipe to remember when you are just about to throw out an over-ripe banana.

1 banana, very ripe

Peel banana and mash well with a fork. Put into small freezer container and freeze, but not too long, maybe about 2 hours. It should be "soft frozen." If it gets really hard you won't be able to eat it.

Per Serving:
Calories: 101 **Fat:** 0g **Carbohydrate:** 26g **Protein:** 1.3g **Sodium:** 0mg

Embarrassingly

Simple

Recipes

Fruit Helper

4 Servings

Packages of mixed dried fruit are available, perfect for this recipe.

> **1 cup mixed dried fruit, cut up**
> **2/3 cup orange juice**
> **1 tablespoon brown sugar**
> **1/2 teaspoon allspice**
> **2 cups applesauce**

Combine all ingredients except applesauce in medium saucepan. Bring to boil. Cover, lower heat, and simmer until mixture starts to thicken, about 5 minutes. (Don't be alarmed that the liquid mostly disappears. It makes the fruit very tender.) Uncover and remove from heat. Put a spoonful on each serving of applesauce.

Per Serving:
Calories: 136   **Fat:** 0g   **Carbohydrate:** 33g   **Protein:** 1g   **Sodium:** 55mg

Warm Winter Fruit

4 Servings

Warm fruit makes a perfect ending to a winter meal. It is also delicious with a brunch buffet.

> 1 8 1/2-ounce can "lite" sliced peaches
> 1 8 1/2-ounce can "lite" pear halves
> 1 8 1/2-ounce can "lite" apricot halves
> 2 tablespoons brown sugar
> 2 teaspoons lemon juice
> 1/2 teaspoon ground cinnamon

Empty cans of fruit, juice and all, into a medium saucepan. Add other ingredients and heat through.

Per Serving:
Calories: 103   **Fat:** 0g   **Carbohydrate:** 26g   **Protein:** 0g   **Sodium:** 15mg

CHAPTER 13

Embarrassingly

Simple

Recipes

Tasty Grapefruit
4 Servings

This is just the thing for those annoying times when, with little or no warning, you have to produce something sort of special.

2 grapefruit, halved and sectioned
4 teaspoons brown sugar

Sprinkle brown sugar over grapefruit halves. Broil 2 inches from heat for 5 minutes, or until golden brown.

Per Serving:
Calories: 28   **Fat:** 0g   **Carbohydrate:** 7g   **Protein:** 0g   **Sodium:** 0g

Hawaiian Pineapple
4 Servings

You can use canned, sliced pineapple for this, but fresh tastes much better. (Hint: try Dole Gold.) Most supermarkets have a device that allows them to peel and core the ripe pineapple for you, which saves you some work at home. Besides dessert, the pineapple makes a nice condiment, particularly with grilled chicken or turkey.

> **4 slices fresh pineapple, peeled, about 1/2-inch thick**
> **OR**
> **4 canned pineapple slices**
> **4 teaspoons honey**

Spread honey on one side only of each pineapple slice. Put on grill, honey side up, and cook for 2 minutes. Flip slices and cook another 2 to 3 minutes.

Per Serving:
Calories: 42   **Fat:** 0g   **Carbohydrate:** 10g   **Protein:** 0g   **Sodium:** 0mg

Embarrassingly

Simple

Recipes

Fresh Berries with Frozen Yogurt and Raspberry Sauce
4 Servings

> 1 pint fresh berries, washed
> 1/2 cup A Great Raspberry Sauce (see recipe, below)
> 1 pint vanilla fat-free frozen yogurt
> 4 sprigs fresh mint (if available)

Using four pretty dishes (dishes can make all the difference), divide berries evenly, put a small scoopful of yogurt on top of berries in each dish, pour raspberry sauce over that, and garnish with mint.

Per Serving:

Calories: 144 **Fat:** 0g **Carbohydrate:** 33g **Protein:** 3g **Sodium:** 67mg

◆   ◆   ◆   ◆

A Great Raspberry Sauce
Makes 1 cup (8 servings)

> 1 10-ounce package frozen raspberries in light syrup, thawed
> 1 tablespoon lemon juice
> 1 tablespoon orange liqueur (optional)

Put raspberries in food processor to purée. Strain to remove seeds if you're feeling ambitious. Add lemon juice; add orange liqueur if desired.

Per Serving:

Calories: 24 **Fat:** 0g **Carbohydrate:** 6g **Protein:** 0g **Sodium:** 0mg

French Toast with a Difference
4 Servings

Looks like breakfast, tastes like breakfast, but why not have it for dessert some cold winter night?

> **1/4 cup egg substitute**
> **1/2 cup fat-free milk**
> **1/2 teaspoon cinnamon**
> **1/4 teaspoon vanilla**
> **4 slices of your favorite bread**
> **All-fruit topping (can be found in the supermarket with the jams and jellies)**

Beat the egg substitute with the milk and cinnamon and vanilla. Soak bread, turning once, and cook in a nonstick skillet until brown. Heat the all-fruit topping over low heat and serve with the french toast.

Per Serving:
Calories: 152   **Fat:** 0g   **Carbohydrate:** 31g   **Protein:** 7g   **Sodium:** 209mg

Embarrassingly

Simple

Recipes

Egg White Omelet *(A fast, delicious, treat)*
Makes one omelet

*Like French Toast with a Difference, this is a breakfast dish that also
makes a wonderful dessert. Keep in mind that it's egg yolks you are trying to avoid, since that's where the fat is. That leaves, by certain calcula-
tions, the whites. (Remember when you made hollandaise sauce and then
tried to figure out what to do with the whites? Now you can use the
whites and try to figure out what to do with the yolks.)*

3 egg whites
2 teaspoons all-fruit jam

Beat egg whites with fork until very fluffy. Spray a small, nonstick skillet lightly with oil, heat, and add egg white mixture. Cook in the hot skillet for 1 minute, turn carefully, and cook other side for 15 to 30 seconds.
Top with all-fruit jam.

Per Omelet:
Calories: 84   **Fat:** 0g   **Carbohydrate:** 11g   **Protein:** 10g   **Sodium:** 150mg

"New Fashioned" Bread Pudding
4 Servings

So called because, unlike the old-fashioned version, this is happily low in fat, while retaining the warm, comforting flavor of the original. It tastes wonderful served warm, which means you don't have to plan all that far ahead.

Notice the recipe calls for stale bread. The slight crispiness keeps it from absorbing too much liquid. If you don't happen to have any stale bread hanging around, you can make your own by laying the slices out on the counter and letting them sit there for awhile, or by very lightly toasting them.

> **1 ½ cups fat-free milk**
> **3/4 cup egg substitute**
> **1/3 cup sugar**
> **1 teaspoon vanilla extract**
> **5 slices stale bread, cut into cubes**

Preheat oven to 350°F.

Mix together all ingredients except bread. Add bread cubes, toss well with "egg" mixture, and pour into 1-quart casserole that has been VERY LIGHTLY sprayed with oil. Bake 1 hour. Allow to cool slightly.

Per Serving:
Calories: 223   **Fat:** 0g   **Carbohydrate:** 44g   **Protein:** 11g   **Sodium:** 145mg

Embarrassingly

Simple

Recipes

Really Nice Custard Dessert
4 Servings

The ingredients are strikingly similar to those in the previous recipe, "New Fashioned" Bread Pudding. Embarrassingly simple recipes are like that.

> 1/4 cup sugar
> 2 cups fat-free milk
> 3/4 cup egg substitute
> 1 teaspoon vanilla
> 1/2 cup fresh berries (optional)

Preheat oven to 350°F.

Rinse a medium saucepan with cold water. (This will keep milk from sticking and make the pot easier to clean.) Combine milk and sugar, then heat almost to boiling, stirring to dissolve the sugar and to make sure you don't scorch the mixture. Remove from heat and gently mix in the egg substitute and the vanilla. Pour into four individual custard cups (oven-proof).

Set in a pan of hot water (or else you'll make four dried-out little cakes instead of custard), and bake for one hour. The custard will seem shivery when it comes out, but it solidifies as it cools. Chill. Top with fresh berries if you wish.

Per Serving:
Calories: 130 **Fat:** 2g **Carbohydrate:** 18g **Protein:** 10g **Sodium:** 146mg

Cherry Cheesecake, Hold the "Cake"
4 Servings

This makes a terrific, romantic dessert because it looks like a Valentine. On the other hand, it "serves 4," and not everyone considers that a romantic number.

1 14 ½-ounce can tart red pitted cherries in water (pie cherries)
1/3 cup sugar
1 tablespoon quick-cooking tapioca

Topping:
1 8-ounce package fat-free cream cheese
2 tablespoons honey
1/4 cup fat-free milk
1/2 teaspoon almond extract

Open can of cherries, measure out 1/2 cup of the juice and put it into a small saucepan, then drain the rest off the cherries. Add sugar and tapioca to the juice, stir, then toss with cherries and allow to stand for a few minutes. Bring cherry mixture to a boil, reduce heat, cover, and simmer for 10 minutes. Remove from heat, uncover, and allow to cool. It will thicken as it cools.

While mixture cools, make topping by blending all topping ingredients in a food processor until smooth. Divide cooled cherries among four dessert dishes and spoon on the topping.

> **SODIUM ALERT!**
> If you are on a sodium-restricted diet, then choose another recipe.

Per Serving:
Calories: 218   **Fat:** 0g   **Carbohydrate:** 43g   **Protein:** 9g   **Sodium:** 410g

Pumpkin Pie-Less (no crust)

8 Servings

1 16-ounce can pumpkin, nothing added
1/2 cup egg substitute
1 teaspoon ground allspice
1/2 teaspoon ground ginger
1/4 teaspoon ground cloves
2/3 cup sugar
1 12-ounce can evaporated skim milk
Nonstick cooking spray

Preheat oven to 400°F.

Combine all ingredients in a large bowl, blend well, and pour into 1-quart casserole dish, LIGHTLY sprayed with oil. Bake for 50 to 60 minutes. May be served warm or at room temperature.

Per Serving:
Calories: 137 **Fat:** 1g **Carbohydrate:** 26g **Protein:** 6g **Sodium:** 86mg

"Chocolate" Birthday Cake
12 Servings

(Made from a mix, of course – and without fat, because we want you to have a lot of birthdays!) This freezes very well.

> **1 box Angel Food Cake mix**
> **1/2 cup unsweetened cocoa powder**

Follow package directions. Before pouring batter into tube pan, add the cocoa powder and blend in well. Continue to follow directions as given on the box.

Per Serving:
Calories: 152 **Fat:** 0g **Carbohydrate:** 33g **Protein:** 5g **Sodium:** 142mg

CHAPTER
13

Embarrassingly

Simple

Recipes

Vanilla Soufflé to Remember
6 Servings

This is the one NON-embarrassingly simple recipe, and has been included because it takes low-fat cooking to new heights. People think that soufflés are difficult to make, and that really isn't true.

When you look at the recipe analysis, you may be surprised to see that there is more fat per serving than we have been recommending, and indeed the recipe calls for 1 1/2 teaspoons rather than one teaspoon of added fat. Otherwise, it follows our rules, incorporating monounsaturated fat (canola oil) and fat-free dairy products (fat-free milk). In addition, by using an egg substitute instead of eggs, a fair amount of fat is eliminated. So – this soufflé becomes a wonderful, special treat, a fine celebration of all your efforts to reduce the fat in your daily diet.

Let's try this together.

Prepare a 2-quart soufflé dish as follows:

Using spray oil, lightly coat the inside of the dish, bottom and sides. Put in a couple of tablespoons of sugar, rotate dish so sugar clings to oil on bottom and sides, and dump out excess.

Now for the soufflé:

> **3 tablespoons canola oil**
> **3 tablespoons flour**
> **1 cup fat-free milk**
> **1/3 cup sugar**
> **1 cup egg substitute**
> **2 teaspoons vanilla**
> **8 egg whites, at room temperature**
> **1 pint fat-free chocolate frozen yogurt, mostly melted**

Preheat oven to 350°F.

Put oil and flour in a saucepan. Using a wire whisk, mix together over moderate heat, stirring constantly. When mixture bubbles, add the milk and sugar. Continue to heat and stir. Lower heat slightly and add egg substitute. DO NOT STOP STIRRING, or you will wind up with something that is so clotted you won't be able to blend it with the egg whites in the next step. Continue to stir until mixture is thickened and smooth. Remove from heat and stir in vanilla. Set aside.

Embarrassingly

Simple

Recipes

Using a large bowl, beat egg whites until stiff but not dry. With an electric mixer this will take several minutes. When you run a rubber spatula through the middle, it should leave a trough. (Another test is that it forms stiff peaks when you pull the spatula up, not little points that sort of fall over.) Pour in the cooled egg substitute mixture and, using that same rubber spatula, fold gently into the whites, so that the air will stay in the egg whites and allow the soufflé to rise impressively. (If you've never folded anything but laundry: With your palm down, keeping the spatula flat against the bowl, pull it along under the mixture and sort of roll it over the top, turning your palm up as you do so. Turn the bowl a bit and repeat. Keep doing this until the yellow egg substitute mixture has combined with the egg whites and the whole thing is a uniform pale yellow. Be gentle as you perform this operation. What you are trying to do is KEEP THE AIR IN THE EGG WHITES.)

Pour into the prepared soufflé dish and bake for about 30 minutes, or until the top is golden brown and dry. (Do not peek during cooking, unless you have one of those ovens with a little window and a light inside.) This is the time for everyone to come and admire, because once you start scooping out the portions with a large serving spoon, the soufflé will begin to collapse. That's fine, though. It will still taste wonderful. Serve with 1/4 cup of the mostly melted frozen yogurt on the side of each plate.

Per Serving:
Calories: 236 **Fat:** 8g **Carbohydrate:** 29g **Protein:** 12g **Sodium:** 194mg

Inspiration

To Keep You On The Low-Fat Track

For Those Moments When You Wonder
How in the World You Got Yourself into This

Remember:

☞ When it comes to low-fat living, you know that any step, no matter how small, is a step in the right direction.

☞ Small, easy steps have *powerful* results.

☞ You are feeling better generally.

☞ You look better, and you may even be shedding some unwanted pounds.

☞ You have taken control of your health in a major way, maybe even extending your life.

☞ You are doing something wonderful for your family – and for yourself.

☞ This is a change **for life**. Can you think of a better reason?

For Further Information

Free! Free! Free! Mostly! An array of publications to help you adapt to low-fat living, including well-designed, colorful pamphlets for the younger generation. Simply send your request(s), along with your name and address, to:

National Heart, Blood and Lung Institute
Information Center
P.O. Box 30105
Bethesda, Maryland 20824-0105
(301) 251-1222

The publications:

"So You Have High Blood Cholesterol"
"Step by Step: Eating to Lower Your High Blood Cholesterol"

For seven- to ten-year-olds:
"Eating with Your Heart in Mind"

For eleven- to fourteen-year-olds:
"Heart Health . . . Your Choice"

For fifteen- to eighteen-year-olds:
"Healthy Heart Habits"

A Parent's Guide:
"Cholesterol in Children: Healthy Eating is a Family Affair"

To get a copy of the Food Guide Pyramid, you can use the mail or the Internet.

Mail: United States Department of Agriculture (USDA)
Center for Nutrition and Public Policy (CNPP)
1120 20th Street NW, Suite 200 N
Washington, DC 20036

Internet: Interactive Food Guide Pyramid
WWW.NAL.USDA.GOV/FNIC/FPYR/PYRAMID.HTML

We want to share with you some of our favorite low-fat cookbooks. You may have to make slight revisions to stay with the four points you now know by heart:

❶ Think 3-ounce serving sizes of Extra Lean meat, fish, or chicken.

❷ Use fat-free or low-fat dairy products.

❸ Use monounsaturated fats, the "fats of choice"– olive and canola oils.

❹ Try to keep recipes near 1 teaspoon added fat per serving.

Jane Brody's Good Food Book, Jane Brody (New York: Bantam Books), 1987.

Jane Brody's Good Food Gourmet, Jane Brody (New York: W.W. Norton & Company), 1992.

Eating Well, Jane Weston Wilson (New York: Workman Publishing), 1987.

Lean Italian Cooking, Anne Casale (New York: Fawcett Columbine), 1994.

The American Heart Association Low-Fat, Low-Cholesterol Cookbook, Scott Grundy and Mary Winston, editors (New York: Random House), 1995.

Other good resources:

"Cooking Light: The Magazine of Food and Fitness," published bimonthly by Southern Living, Inc.
Call (800) 336-0125 for subscription information.

"Nutrition Action Healthletter," published monthly by the Center for Science in the Public Interest
1875 Connecticut Avenue, N.W.
Suite 300
Washington, DC 20009-5728
Or call (202) 332-9110 for subscription information.

Endnotes

1. Several important studies in the last fifteen years have identified a fatty substance in the blood that is associated with heart disease, and is called – you guessed it – cholesterol. However, in and of itself it is not a villain, but is an integral part of animal cell structure and a major component of brain tissue. In other words, without cholesterol we would be cell-less and brain-less. Cholesterol is so important that the liver produces what the body needs. (page 18)

2. Jane Brody, *Jane Brody's New York Times Guide to Personal Health* (New York: Times Books), 1982, p. 24. (page 19)

3. K.L. Gould, D. Ornish, L. Scherwitz, et al., "Changes in Myocardial Perfusion Abnormalities by Positron Emission Tomography After Long-Term, Intense Risk Factor Modification," *Journal of the American Medical Association*, 274(11):894-901, 1995. (page 19)

4. High-fat diets tend to increase "insulin resistance," which predisposes a person to diabetes. The very newest research is examining the connection between insulin resistance and heart disease. (page 19)

    E.J. Mayer-Davis, J.H. Monaco, H.M. Hoen, et al., "Dietary Fat and Insulin Sensitivity in a Triethnic Population: The Role of Obesity. The Insulin Resistance Atherosclerosis Study (IRAS)," *American Journal of Clinical Nutrition*, 65:79-87, 1997.

5. L.J. Appel, T.J. Moore, E. Obarzanek, et al., "A Clinical Trial of the Effects of Dietary Patterns on Blood Pressure," *New England Journal of Medicine*, 336(16):1117-24, 1997. (page 19)

6. How do you know if you're eating a lot of sugar? Sugars can be found in various disguises, so check the Ingredient List for any of these obvious sugars – corn syrup, molasses, honey, brown sugar – as well as these less obvious ones: glucose, sucrose, fructose, levulose, maltose, whey, mannitol, and sorbitol.

   There are no studies that show that sugar causes heart disease (just cavities). But while it can't hurt, it doesn't help. Sugar contains no vitamins, minerals, or fiber, and by taking in energy in the form of sugar, you tend not to eat foods that are good for you: fruits, vegetables, and starches. (page 29)

7. Nutrition Labeling and Education Act of 1990. *Federal Register*, 58(3): 654, 1993. (page 30)

8. "Beans, Beans, the musical fruit,
   The more you eat, the more you toot.
   The more you toot, the better you feel,
   So eat baked beans at every meal." (page 30)

9. Rinsing canned beans before using them, or soaking dried beans and discarding that water before cooking them in fresh water, will help decrease flatulence. (page 31)

10. Starchy beans, as well as oats and barley, contain soluble fiber, which lowers serum cholesterol levels. (page 31)

    P.B. Geil, J.W. Anderson, "Dry Beans: Nutrition Implications," *Journal of the American College of Nutrition*, 13(6): 549-58, 1994.

    D.J.A. Jenkins, T.M.S. Wolever, A.V. Rao, et al., "Effect on Blood Lipids of Very High Intakes of Fiber in Diets Low in Saturated Fat and Cholesterol," *New England Journal of Medicine*, 329:21-6, 1993.

11. Current research shows that fruits and vegetables contain thousands of

compounds, many of which are only now beginning to be studied. While there is still a pleasant mystery to the whole thing, we do know that fruits and vegetables pack a health wallop, and that it is far better to eat these foods than it is to take vitamin and mineral supplements. (page 32)

12. S.M. Krebs-Smith, A. Cook, A.F. Subar, "U.S. Adults' Fruit and Vegetable Intakes, 1989 to 1991: A Revised Baseline for the *Healthy People 2000* Objective," *American Journal of Public Health*, 85(12): 1623-29, 1995. (page 32)

13. *Vegetables and Specialties: Situation and Outlook Yearbook*. U.S. Dept. of Agriculture, Economic Research Service: 9, 1992. (page 32)

14. It doesn't take much protein to make new cells, et cetera, and most people eat more than they need. Unless you have a specific medical reason, you do not need to worry about eating too little protein. (If you are concerned that you have special protein needs, seek professional advice.) As long as you eat a wide variety of starches and vegetables, you'll be getting plenty of protein, and you'll be eating less fat. (page 39)

15. V. Fonnebo, "Mortality in Norwegian Seventh-Day Adventists 1962-1986," *Journal of Clinical Epidemiology*, 45(2):157-67, 1992. (page 39)

M. Kestin and I.L. Rouse, "Cardiovascular Disease Risk Factors in Free-Living Men: Comparison of Two Prudent Diets, One Based on Lactoovovegetarianism and the other allowing Lean Meat," *American Journal of Clinical Nutrition*," 50(2):280-87, 1989.

16. M.L. Daviglus, J. Stamler, A.J. Orencia, et al., "Fish Consumption and the 30-year Risk of Fatal Myocardial Infarction," *New England Journal of Medicine*, 336(15): 1046-53, 1997.

M.L. Burr, A.M. Fehily, J.F. Gilbert, et al., "Effects of Changes in Fat,

Fish, and Fibre Intakes on Death and Myocardial Reinfarction: Diet and Reinfarction Trial (DART)," *Lancet,* 334:757-61, 1989. (page 43)

17. Even though shellfish is very, very low in fat, it does not qualify as "extra lean" or "lean" because it contains too much cholesterol to qualify. But don't be fooled by the name. The "cholesterol" in shellfish seems to be different, maybe even beneficial. (page 43)

M.T. Childs, C.S. Dorsett, A. Failor, et al., "Effect of Shellfish Consumption on Cholesterol Absorption in Normolipidemic Men," *Metabolism: Clinical and Experimental*, 36(1):31-35, 1987.

18. If you decide to give up high-fat cheese, don't throw out the baby with the bath water. You still need a source of calcium, which you can get from low-fat and fat-free dairy products. Without them, you probably need calcium supplements. Check with a doctor or registered dietitian. (page 43)

19. Well-planned, complete meals can lower cholesterol levels. This study was done with pre-packaged meals. (page 48)

D.A. McCarron, S. Oparil, A. Chait, et al., "Nutritional Management of Cardiovascular Risk Factors," *Archives of Internal Medicine*, 157:169-177, 1997.

20. The Lyon Diet Heart Study showed 70% reduction in heart attacks and cardiac deaths among individuals who consumed a Mediterranean-type diet. They ate more bread, more root vegetables and green vegetables, more fish, and less meat than usual, and they ate fruit every day. The fat they used was monounsaturated. (page 52)

M. de Lorgeril, S. Renaud, N. Mamelle, et al., "Mediterranean Alpha-Linolenic Acid-Rich Diet in Secondary Prevention of Coronary Heart Disease," *Lancet*, 343:1454-59, 1994.

21. This means that there is no protein and no carbohydrate in margarine. All the calories come from fat. Even if it is a reduced-calorie version, there are simply fewer calories, but they all come from fat. (page 54)

22. Consumption of partially hydrogenated vegetable oils (it's that *trans* fat) may contribute to coronary heart disease. (page 54)

    W. Willett, M. Stampfer, J. Mason, et al., "Intake of *Trans* Fatty Acids and Risk of Coronary Heart Disease Among Women," *Lancet*, 341:581-85, 1993.

    For a review of the literature:
    W. Willet and A. Ascherio, "*Trans* Fatty Acids: Are the Effects Only Marginal?" *American Journal of Public Health*, 84:722-24, 1994.

23. Here's how we've arrived at those 65 grams:
    1 teaspoon of fat = 5 grams
    13 teaspoons of fat = 65 grams
        That is, 13 x 5 = 65

    Incidentally:
        1 gram of fat = 9 calories
        65 grams of fat = 585 calories
        (That is, 65 x 9 = 585)   (page 60)

24. When you saw that little number, you thought we were going to list the "many, many texts available on the subject," didn't you?
    Instead, we'll make one suggestion. Like the other texts, this comes complete with charts that will help you determine "your daily fat-grams budget," as this book calls it. Joseph Piscatella, *Choices for A Healthy Heart* (New York: Workman Publishing), 1987. (page 61)

25. "Physical Activity and Cardiovascular Health" (pamphlet), *National Institutes of Health Consensus Statement*, 13(3), 1995. (page 61)

26. Fantastic Foods "Only a Pinch" is a low-sodium dehydrated soup. Check labels for others. (page 94)

27. For more information about introducing new foods to children, see: Ellyn Satter, *How to Get Your Kid to Eat . . . But Not Too Much* (Palo Alto, CA: Bull Publishing Co.), 1987. (page 101)

28. Rosemary Tindle, "Home Economist Notes…Fried Turkeys," *Tunica Times*, Tunica, Mississippi, 12/19/96. (page 103)

29. This and other statements in this chapter ("Foods Your Heart Will Love") are supported by numerous studies published in such respected research journals as *The New England Journal of Medicine*, *Journal of the American Medical Association, Lancet*, and *Journal of Nutrition*, among others. We've included one study from each section, a sample of just what we mean. If you want more of the same, e-mail us at: realpple@erols.com

HOMOCYSTEINE:
C.J. Boushey, S.A. Beresford, G.S. Omenn, et al., "A Quantitative Assessment of Plasma Homocysteine as a Risk Factor for Vascular Disease," *Journal of the American Medical Association*, 274(13): 1049-57, 1995.

OATS:
C.M. Ripsin, J.M. Keenan, D.R. Jacobs, et al., "Oat Products and Lipid Lowering, a Meta-Analysis," *Journal of the American Medical Association*, 267(24):3317-25, 1992.

SOY:
J.W. Anderson, B.M. Johnstone, M.E. Cook-Newell, "Meta-Analysis of the Effects of Soy Protein Intake on Serum Lipids," *New England Journal of Medicine*, 333(5):276-82, 1995.

GARLIC:

S. Warshafsky, R.S. Kamer, S.L Sivak, "Effect of Garlic on Total Cholesterol, A Meta-analysis," *Annals of Internal Medicine*, 119:599-605, 1993.

NUTS:

M.L. Dreher and C.V Maher, "The Traditional and Emerging Role of Nuts in Healthful Diets," *Nutrition Reviews*, 54(8): 241-45, 1996.

K.J.A. Jenkins, D.G. Popovich, C.W.C. Kendall, et al., "Effect of a Diet High in Vegetables, Fruit and Nuts on Serum Lipids," *Metabolism: Clinical and Experimental*, 46:530-37, 1997.

VITAMIN E:

N.G. Stephens, A. Parsons, Peter M. Schofield, et al, "Randomised Controlled Trial of Vitamin E in Patients with Coronary Disease: Cambridge Heart Antioxidant Study (CHAOS)," *Lancet*, 347:781-86, 1996.

    The "CHAOS" study. You've gotta love the name. (page 115)

30. If you're taking a pure folic acid supplement, check with your doctor to make sure you do not have a vitamin B-12 deficiency. (page 115)

31. Effects were more pronounced for those with cholesterol levels above 229 than for those with levels below that. (page 117)

32. This trivia is brought to you by an out-of-print book:
Dorothea Van Gundy Jones, *The Soybean Cookbook (New York:* Arco Publishing Co., Inc), 1974, p. 5. (page 119)

33. There's convincing evidence that soy protein lowers cholesterol as much as 9% in people with high cholesterol levels. So how much, exactly, is enough to do the job? Well, the jury is still out on that one. In thirty-eight studies, the soy protein consumed averaged 47

grams per day, but that is not a recommended amount. As of this writing, there is no recommended amount. Discussion continues. If you want to know how many grams of protein are found in each product, here's a handy reference:

PRODUCT	SERVING	GRAMS OF PROTEIN
ISP	1/4 cup	13-23
Soy beans (fresh)	3 ounces	10
Soy milk	1 cup	4-10
Tofu	4 ounces	13
TSP	1 cup	22

Above information comes from Anne Patterson, "Now That Soy Protein Has Respect, How Do You Eat More?", *Soy Connection*, 4(1):3, 1996. (page 119)

34. ISP = Isolated Soy Protein
    TSP = Texturized Soy Protein (page 119)

35. Use of garlic lowered cholesterol an average of 9%. Studies used one to three cloves of garlic, or else 600-900 mg of garlic powder preparations a day. Note, however, that these studies are only preliminary, and there are as yet no actual recommendations. (page 120)

36. People who ate nuts 1-4 times a week had 25% reduced risk of heart disease. People who ate nuts 5 or more times a week had 50% reduced risk. (page 121)

37. Terms on labels that are useful in helping you eat less fat:

    "Fat Free"– less than 0.5g total fat per serving.

    "Low Fat"– 3g or less total fat per serving. ("Low Fat" may not be a bargain if their serving size is only two crackers. Again, check your OPSS.)

"Extra Lean"– no more than 5 grams of total fat, 2 grams of saturated fat, in a 3-ounce serving.

"Lean"– no more than 10 grams of total fat, 4.5 grams of saturated fat, in a 3-ounce serving.

CHECK LABELS FURTHER BEFORE ASSUMING LOW TOTAL FAT.

"Low Saturated Fat"– 1g or less saturated fat per serving. *Does not necessarily mean the product is low in total fat.*

"Less Fat," "Reduced Fat"– 25 percent less total fat than the original version. (It may be worth taking a look at the original version, which might be so high in fat that a 25 percent reduction still leaves an awful lot in there.)

"Light"– contains 1/3 the calories or 1/2 the fat of the original version of the food. Technically a product can be called "light" by reducing calories only, which still leaves the product with the original amount of fat. Also, you can have a "light" product with 50 percent fat. As an example, margarine is 100 percent fat and can be called "light" if its fat content is reduced by 50 percent (the other 50 percent is air). It's still all fat, though.

"Low Cholesterol"– less than 20mg per serving, and less than 2g saturated fat per serving. You could still be eating a high-fat product. *"Low cholesterol" does not mean low fat.* (page 124)

38. Wayne Gisslen, *Professional Cooking* (New York: John Wiley and Sons), 1983, p. 318. (page 127)

39. "Single ingredient raw foods" include fresh produce, raw fish, meat, and poultry. Labeling on these foods is strictly voluntary, but who needs labels on fresh fruits and vegetables anyway? Meat and poultry are a different story altogether. We need specific information for

each cut of meat. Nutrition information is probably somewhere in the store, but it may be hard to get. Too bad. We need it. (page 132)

40. Here is some general comparative information about the fat content of various lunch meats, cheeses, and mayonnaise-based salads.

    As far as lunch meats go, your first choice is, of course, those that say "fat free" or "low fat" right on the package. Beyond that, different brands of lunch meat contain slightly different amounts of fat, but this will give you a good idea of what you're dealing with. Remember, you are looking for Extra Lean and Lean meats.

Product	Serving size	Amount of fat
Turkey breast	two slices (two ounces)	2.0g
Ham (extra lean)	"	2.8g
Bologna	"	6.5g
Turkey salami	"	6.8g
Regular salami	"	10.0g

Pretty thin sandwich you have there. Are you sure you eat only two slices? Think OPSS (Own Personal Serving Size).

Cheeses are another question altogether. We can tell you how much fat is in an ounce of a given cheese, but then again, you think of eating a *piece* of cheese, not an ounce of cheese, so you're probably wondering what that one ounce looks like. Was it cut from a brick of cheese? A wedge? Is it prepackaged, with those little pieces of paper in between the slices? Is it sliced at the deli counter, so that a piece of Swiss is approximately the size of a notepad? And how about grated cheese? The next time you're at the supermarket, treat yourself to an ounce of a number of different shaped cheeses, and you'll begin to get used to what an ounce looks like.

Product	Serving size	Amount of fat
Mozzarella	one ounce	7g
Parmesan	"	7g
Swiss	"	8g
American	"	9g
Cheddar	"	9g

As you can see, cheese is high in fat, so if you are determined to eat a lot of it, you might want to examine high-tech cheeses, on which the terms "fat free" or "low fat" will surely appear. Manufacturers have managed to take all or some of the fat out of them, but you are likely to find that the taste has also been taken out, and when you try to heat the cheese, you are left with something that looks as if it should be played with rather than eaten.

Mayonnaise-based products: Note that one ounce of these salads is only about 1/8 cup. Chances are that you eat more than that, probably at least half a cup, which contains 4 times the fat that is listed here. That is, an average serving of one of these salads would contain about 16 grams of fat.

Product	Serving size	Amount of fat
Potato salad	one ounce	3.0g
Chicken salad	"	4.0g
Macaroni salad	"	4.0g
Ham salad	"	4.5g

Meat information is based on J. Pope-Cordle and M. Katahn, *The Low-Fat Supermarket Shopper's Guide* (New York: W.W. Norton and Company, New York), 1993, and J. Pennington, *Bowes and Church's Food Values of Portions Commonly Used*, 16th ed. (Philadelphia, PA: J.B. Lippincott Company), 1994.

Cheese information is based on *Bowes and Church's Food Values of Portions Commonly Used*, above.

Salad information is based on J. Pope-Cordle and M. Katahn, *The T-Factor Fat Gram Counter* (New York: W.W. Norton and Company), 1991, and *Bowes and Church's Food Values of Portions Commonly Used*, above. (page 132)

41. *Current Medical Diagnosis and Treatment*, 1997 Edition, edited by L.M. Tierney, Jr., S.J. McPhee, and M.A. Papadakis, p. 1124. (page 135)

42. Angiographic studies ("up close and personal" looks inside the arteries) show that a low-fat diet decreases the amount of plaque ("gunk") in the arteries of the heart. The lower the total fat in the diet, the greater the improvement.

     In the STARS study, a 27 percent-fat diet was followed. Plaque decreased in 38 percent of the participants.
     G.F. Watts, P. Jackson, S. Mandalia, et al., "Nutrient Intake and Progression of Coronary Artery Disease," *American Journal of Cardiology*, 73: 328-32, 1994.

     In the Lifestyle Heart Study, conducted by Dean Ornish, participants followed a 10 percent-fat diet; arterial plaque decreased in 82 percent of the individuals studied.
     D. Ornish, S.E. Brown, Z.W. Scherwitz, et al., "Can Lifestyle Changes Reverse Coronary Heart Disease? The Lifestyle Heart Trial," *Lancet*, 336:129-33, 1990. (page 135)

43. The "Embarrassingly Simple Recipes" stay within government guidelines for heart-healthy foods (*Federal Register*, pp. 2494-95):

	Single Food	**Main Dish**
Total Fat (g)	13	19.5
Saturated Fat (g)	4	6
Cholesterol (mg)	60	90
Sodium (mg)	480	720

     Exceptions are shrimp (Shrimp with Tomatoes) and pink salmon (Crunchy Tuna Salad made with salmon); both are higher in cholesterol than suggested in the guidelines. We have included them because other aspects of all seafood and fish make them fine additions to a heart-healthy diet. (page 139)

Index

Here's what they're saying about
Low-Fat Living for Real People...

"...offers readers comprehensive yet 'embarrassingly simple' how-to strategies for adopting a heart-healthy diet ... uncluttered with hype ... has the potential to significantly improve health."

> *Penny Kris-Etherton, Ph.D., R.D.*
> *Distinguished Professor of Nutrition*
> *Pennsylvania State University*

"Let's get total fat down. Use this helpful book to start on a low-fat diet now!"

> *Paul A. LaChance, Ph.D.*
> *Professor of Food Science and Nutrition*
> *Rutgers University*

"Very useful, easy to read, and humorous, as well."

> *Susan C. Brozena, M.D.*
> *Medical Director,*
> *Heart Failure/Transplant Center*
> *Allegheny University Hospital*
> *Philadelphia, PA*

"The simplicity of these recipes is very appealing."

> *Ceri Hadda*
> *Food writer and author,* Coffee Cakes